OXFORD MEDICAL PUBLICATIONS

World Blindness
and its Prevention

Volume 3

World Blindness and its Prevention

Volume 3

Edited by
the International Agency for the Prevention of Blindness
under the direction of Carl Kupfer, MD

The IAPB wishes to acknowledge the contribution made by
Terrence Gillen, MA, MBA, to the compilation and
editing of this book

Oxford New York Melbourne
OXFORD UNIVERSITY PRESS
1988

Oxford University Press, Walton Street, Oxford OX2 6DP
Oxford   New York   Toronto
Delhi   Bombay   Calcutta   Madras   Karachi
Petaling Jaya   Singapore   Hong Kong   Tokyo
Nairobi   Dar es Salaam   Cape Town
Melbourne   Auckland
and associated companies in
Berlin   Ibadan

Oxford is a trade mark of Oxford University Press

Published in the United States
by Oxford University Press, New York

British Library Cataloguing in Publication Data
World blindness and its prevention.
Vol. 3
1. Man. Blindness. Prevention
I. Kupfer, Carl   II. International Agency
for the Prevention of Blindness
617.7'12
ISBN 0-19-261755-9

Library of Congress Cataloging in Publication Data
(Revised for volume 3)
World blindness and its prevention.
(Oxford medical publications)
GB80
Vol. 3-   edited under the direction of Carl Kupfer.
Chiefly papers presented at meetings of the General Assembly of the
International Agency for the Prevention of Blindness.
Includes index.
1. Blindness——Prevention——Congresses.   I. Wilson, John, Sir, 1919-   .
II. Kuper, Carl, 1928-   .
III. International Agency for the Prevention of Blindness. General Assembly.
RE91.W67   617.7'12052   79-41190
ISBN 0-19-261249-2 (v. 1)
0-19-261755-9 (vol. 3)

Set by Colset Private Limited, Singapore
Printed in Great Britain
at the University Printing House, Oxford
by David Stanford
Printer to the University

At least half of all blindness in the world is preventable. The International Agency for the Prevention of Blindness (IAPB), with its national and international partners, seeks to reduce the global toll of 40 million blind people by increasing awareness of this problem among the people of the world and their governments, by encouraging financial and manpower support of blindness prevention programmes, and by promoting the development of effective prevention programmes employing the most appropriate and economic technology.

Preface

Over 400 ophthalmologists, eye care professionals, public health specialists, managers, and others engaged in the battle against avoidable blindness attended the Third General Assembly of the International Agency for the Prevention of Blindness (IAPB) in New Delhi, India, from 6 to 11 December 1986. The IAPB is a multinational, world-wide consortium of groups and individuals committed to reducing the global toll of blindness. The IAPB evaluates needs and opportunities for the prevention of blindness, primarily in developing countries, and seeks to expedite the development of strong programmes and to co-ordinate the availability of necessary resources. Currently, 64 national prevention of blindness committees participate in the activities of the Agency. In addition, the World Health Organization (WHO) co-operates in the efforts of the IAPB—especially helping to mobilize resources and political will—as do a number of international voluntary and philanthropic organizations.

The theme of the meeting, 'A Decade of Progress', coincided with the completion of 10 years of world-wide IAPB service. The First General Assembly was held in 1978 in Oxford, England; the Second was in Bethesda, Maryland, United States, in 1982. At the Third General Assembly we had the opportunity to gather in India's uniquely instructive and inspiring setting. The selection of this country as the site of this meeting is highly significant. In India we see both the problem of avoidable blindness and the means of combating it displayed on a massive scale. This nation endures a formidable toll of visual loss each year, yet she is doing something about this problem through highly effective programmes that have won wide support within the country and internationally. This General Assembly was jointly sponsored by the Indian National Society for the Prevention of Blindness and the Times (of India) Eye Research Foundation.

In those who attended the Third General Assembly were all the key ingredients of IAPB's success over the past decade and a great wealth of experience and determination acquired through years of successful efforts against blindness. There were representatives of the World Health Organization and the major non-governmental organizations for the prevention of blindness. In addition, there were representatives from ministries of health and national IAPB

committees for the prevention of blindness, and eye care professionals who have dedicated their own skills to this great cause. These
dedicated people used the Third General Assembly to share their
experiences, to learn valuable lessons from the many successful
programmes that were discussed, and to strengthen each other's
resolve to continue the battle against avoidable blindness. This
book presents the most salient materials gathered for and presented
at this General Assembly.

Bethesda, Maryland   C.K.
January 1988

Message to the Third General Assembly of the IAPB

H. Mahler, Director-General, World Health Organization

It gives me great pleasure to send a message to the Third General Assembly of the International Agency for the Prevention of Blindness.

The Agency has now completed its first decade of successful action for the prevention of blindness throughout the world. The IAPB has, indeed, become instrumental in the promotion of the concept of avoidable blindness, particularly in developing countries and through the rapidly increasing number of its national committees.

The history of your Agency is closely related to that of the World Health Organization and the establishment of our Programme for the Prevention of Blindness. We can look back at a decade of very rewarding collaboration in this field, and we shall develop this further in our joint efforts for 'Health for All by the Year 2000'. The important role that non-governmental organizations can play in support of strategies to attain this goal was highlighted during the Technical Discussions of the Thirty-eighth World Health Assembly in 1985. The International Agency for the Prevention of Blindness has already taken on the task of mobilizing the community of non-governmental organizations working in the field of blindness prevention to join in the efforts of the World Health Organization and its Blindness Programme. The rapidly increasing number of national programmes for the prevention of blindness—at present in some 50 countries—bears witness to the effectiveness of bringing non-governmental organizations into the framework of the World Health Organization's technical co-operation with its Member States. Furthermore, the unanimous support by the International Agency, its member organizations, and its committees to the primary health care approach to the prevention of blindness developed within the WHO Programme has proved extremely valuable in facilitating the rapid implementation of numerous projects for eye care at the community level.

As the year 2000 approaches, our continued efforts are needed to make the goal of 'Health for All by the Year 2000' a reality. Much work has been done in the field of preventing unnecessary visual loss, but much also remains to be done. I am convinced that this, the Third General Assembly of the International Agency for the Prevention of Blindness, will contribute significantly to the expansion of blindness prevention activities to areas and populations not yet involved, and in finding ways of mobilizing the further resources needed for work in this field.

I wish this Assembly every success in its deliberations.

Contents

Contributors

Chandler R. Dawson,

Director, Francis I, Proctor Foundation for Research in Ophthalmology, University of California, San Francisco, California, USA.

Sally Deitz,

National Consultant on Low Vision, The American Foundation for the Blind, New York, New York, USA.

Michael F. Drummond,

Director, Health Services Management Centre, University of Birmingham, UK.

Leon B. Ellwein,

Professor and Associate Dean, University of Nebraska Medical Centre, Omaha, Nebraska, USA.

Eva Friedlander,

Senior Research Associate, The American Foundation for the Blind, New York, New York, USA.

Carl Kupfer,

President, IAPB and Director, National Eye Institute, National Institutes of Health, Bethesda, Maryland, USA.

Hugh R. Taylor,

Associate Director, The International Centre for Epidemiology and Preventive Ophthalmology, The Wilmer Institute, The Johns Hopkins University, Baltimore, Maryland, USA.

Bjorn Thylefors,

Programme Manager, Prevention of Blindness, World Health Organization, Geneva, Switzerland.

Barbara A. Underwood,

Special Assistant for Nutrition Research and International Programmes, National Eye Institute, National Institutes of Health,
Bethesda, Maryland, USA.

Randolph Whitfield Jr.,

Royal Commonwealth Society for the Blind and Operation Eyesight
Universal, Mt. Kenya Estates, Nyeri, Kenya.

Sir John Wilson,

(Honorary President, IAPB), Impact, 22 The Cliff, Roedean,
Brighton, East Sussex, UK.

1

Preventing blindness, a retrospective

Sir John Wilson
Honorary President, IAPB

It is astonishing how ancient are some of the technologies for the
relief of disability. The Greeks and Romans had hearing aids. Medi-
eval armourers made articulated artificial limbs. Two thousand
years ago, in Southern India, eye doctors were removing cataracts.

Wall-paintings in Egyptian pyramids show sophisticated dis-
crimination between different eye diseases. The tenth-century
medical school in Baghdad had what today would be called a
department of ophthalmology.

The prevention of disability, particularly blindness, deafness, and
orthopaedic impairment, was one of the preoccupations of early
medicine. It was something about which scientists speculated, phi-
losophers philosophized, and saints prayed.

In those early days the prevalence of blindness in all countries
must have been at least as great as it is today in the most under-
served communities. However, it is probably only in modern times—
with the development of great conurbations with multi-million
populations, disease transferring communications, and increasing
longevity—that the number of blind people in the world has
increased to tens of millions. At the same time, the science of
ophthalmology has developed as a distinct discipline and the great
ophthalmic hospitals and research institutions have stimulated the
advance of visual sciences to the point where they now constitute
one of the most successful applications of remedial medicine.

In all these years, there have been remarkable individual pioneers,
who developed institutions and concepts well ahead of their time.
The first prevention of blindness societies were established in
London in 1882 and in New York in 1908. In 1929 the International
Association for the Prevention of Blindness was formed within the
International Congress of Ophthalmology.

The International Agency, formed in 1974, owed much to the
work of the former International Association and to the Prevention
of Blindness Committee of the World Council for the Welfare of the
Blind. It was the coming together of these two organizations, and
their alliance with the World Health Organization (WHO), which

created the Agency and saw its task in terms of community eye care, appropriate technology, multi-disciplinary co-operation and a combination of the technical skills of the ophthalmic profession, the promotional talent of the organizations for the blind, and the advocacy and commitment of blind people themselves.

At the first European Congress of Ophthalmology, in Athens in 1960, Sir Stuart Duke-Elder and I proposed co-operation between ophthalmologists and blind welfare workers. At a meeting in Jerusalem, organized by Professor Michaelson, the concept was formulated of a Global Programme for the Prevention of Blindness. At that meeting were many of the people who later took the initiative in creating that Programme.

Meetings of the World Health Assembly, concerned initially with trachoma and onchocerciasis, gradually expanded WHO's concern into a comprehensive programme. At the World Health Assembly in 1972, a resolution was adopted to consolidate the advance towards a global programme. The prevention of blindness was the theme of two World Health Days, which did much to bring the facts to international attention.

At the outset the case for action was inhibited by grossly inadequate statistics based often on census returns that enumerated only the totally blind. In the 1950s, surveys conducted by the Royal Commonwealth Society for the Blind revealed, for the first time, communities where over 1 per cent of the population was blind. However, as late as 1970, official doubts were expressed about the preliminary estimate that there might be 16 million blind people in the world.

One difficulty was the definition of blindness. An official questionnaire revealed over 70 different definitions in use in UN member states. Eventually, an expert committee, not without considerable debate, formulated the standard scale of visual acuity. On the basis of that scale in 1978, a WHO Task Force estimated that, according to which of two points was adopted on that scale, there were likely to be from 28 million to 42 million blind people in the world.

An inter-regional committee in Baghdad agreed that the priorities of the Global Programme should be what were then called the 'four giants': onchocerciasis, trachoma, xerophthalmia, and cataract. Those priorities were formulated against a considerable swell of opposition. Purists in WHO maintained that cataract, being curable and not preventable, should not logically be part of the Programme. There was similar controversy about including xerophthalmia, on the grounds that to include it as a specific part of the prevention of blindness programme might deflect from the generality of the movement towards primary health. That reservation disappeared during the Bangladesh famine winter of 1972, when world opinion was faced with the appalling prospect of scores of thousands of infants blinded by vitamin A deficiency.

The Global Programme benefited from the climate of optimism created by the eradication of smallpox. Subsequent progress is charted in the Minutes of WHO's Advisory Group. That Group owes much to the programme managers and to its outstanding membership, drawing inter-regionally on authoritative advice from leading ophthalmologists, research workers, and administrators.

In this whole perspective it would be difficult to exaggerate the importance of the Indian National Programme. With the patronage and personal interest of Mrs Indira Gandhi, and the administrative thrust of national and state ministries of health, it provided a convincing demonstration of what can be done in a national programme that has the support of an enlightened government. That programme, and work throughout South-East Asia, owed much also to the stimulus of WHO's Regional Office in New Delhi.

The first priority of the International Agency for the Prevention of Blindness was the establishment of national committees as the nucleus of national programmes. These committees, some covering a vast and complex area such as the Soviet Union and others concerned with a small community such as a West Indian island, formulated national plans and laid the foundation for effective collaboration between government and the private sector.

The search for appropriate technology also owed much to the Indian subcontinent. 'Eye camps' had been developed many years earlier in India and Pakistan but the problem was to maintain quality and to combine the improvisation and community involvement of the village with professionally acceptable standards of surgery and aftercare. This was achieved by the practical dedication of some of the leaders of rural ophthalmology in India, who were prepared to see their hospital not as a static centre of exclusive treatment but as a focal point of a rural programme with mobile teams achieving genuine community involvement. In 1969, the Royal Commonwealth Society for the Blind launched the 'Eyes of India' campaign, with its emphasis on cataract and xerophthalmia and involving many of the leading hospitals and voluntary organizations throughout the subcontinent. That campaign, by establishing procedures for mass treatment in rural areas, helped to make eye camps professionally respectable and led to the Indian National Programme.

Regional and national programmes followed rapidly in the

Western Pacific, the Middle East, Africa, and Latin America. From Europe, North America, the Soviet Union, Japan, and Oceania, notable technical resources were mobilized. The consortium of non-governmental organizations was formed and WHO, in different countries, identified collaborating centres for strategy, research, and staff training.

The World Congress of Ophthalmology and the regional academies began to give priority on their agendas to the prevention of blindness. In many countries, organizations of and for the blind added, to their traditional role of rehabilitation, real concern for the conservation of sight.

The concept of eye care as an essential component of primary health developed during this period as a practical and obtainable contribution to WHO's strategy of Health for All. The West-African Onchocerciasis Control Programme, achieved results that may well rank with smallpox as one of the most successful medical interventions of the second half of this century. Xerophthalmia, originally seen as an unpronounceable medical curiosity, advanced to the point where WHO could launch a global programme of control. Successful interventions against cataract opened the prospect of a world effort to clear the backlog of curable blindness.

Inevitably, as the organization and its conceptual framework expanded, there were differences of opinion about priority, strategy, professional, and administrative boundaries. These differences have never been a serious brake on the programme and, although much remains to be done, the progress which has been achieved has exceeded expectation. This has been particularly so during the past four years, with vigorous management in Geneva, with the invaluable commitment of the international non-governmental organizations and with outstanding professional leadership. Perhaps the best testimony to the success of this programme is that it is increasingly seen as a model of non-governmental co-operation and as the prototype for the international initiative that is now developing against avoidable disability.

2

Inaugural address, Third General Assembly

Shri Rajiv Gandhi
Prime Minister, India

Traditionally, in India we have not treated blindness as a handicap to work. Perhaps I can best illustrate that by going back to the story of one of our legendary kings, Drutharashtra, who was blind. He ruled well for many years until he was asked to decide which two branches of his family should succeed him. The Pandavas had the legitimate right and the Kavaravas were the usurpers. Although he had ruled well for many years, he said he could not make the decision between the two because he was blind. In India we do not consider physical blindness a handicap but only moral blindness—which is a much bigger malady. Traditionally, the only sin in India is the sin of Drutharashtra.

We feel in India it is not enough to attempt to solve problems at the macro level—trying to get an overall view. This is especially true in attempting the development and building of a nation. We believe that it is equally important to go down to the individual human being because we know that there is no true national development possible unless we can reach out into the life of every person.

Perhaps this dual approach has lead to blindness being considered such an important problem in India. One of the first things I did after winning the election was to organize a series of eye camps that included the whole mix from prevention to treatment. Those were probably the most successful programmes that we have undertaken, and they were broadened from just a few constituencies at first to include eventually the whole country.

Although there were a few problems, we found that by and large the infection rate has been no worse in the eye camps than in the hospitals. Perhaps the doctors are more careful in the camps because they understand the shortcomings that are a natural part of working under those conditions. Perhaps the surgeons' extra care has made up for the lack of facilities. Nevertheless, we will persevere to improve and continue this programme.

In India, blindness affects a fairly large number of people, especially those who are poor. The problem cannot be separated by

5

political boundaries. It is a human problem and in attempting to prevent blindness, even more than in other fields, we must all work together. Primarily because of the thrust Indira Gandhi gave to the prevention of blindness programme, India has made substantial accomplishments in supplementing nutrition and in providing nutrition education. Through these two programmes we have reduced the nutrition-related causes of blindness to less than 2 per cent.

Indira Gandhi's 20-point programme has accentuated the prevention of blindness. In addition, cataract operations over the past five years have restored sight to more than five million people and anti-glaucoma programmes have greatly reduced glaucoma-related blindness. But in developing countries it is perhaps more important to prevent blindness, and to take preventive measures at very early stages, than it is to concentrate on curing existing diseases. This is true primarily because the investment in prevention gives us a much better chance to save sight.

We have targeted to reduce the blindness rate in India from 1.5 to 0.3 per cent by the year 2000. This very large reduction will be realized through the use of public health facilities, primary health centres, mobile units, eye camps, and—perhaps most significantly— through voluntary agencies. We hope that as a result of this international meeting there will be more steps taken against blinding eye diseases, not just in India but throughout the world.

We have taken a number of steps to use the media, but I believe that public-service messages are not the answer because people tend to switch off their sets when these begin. However, we have had success with televised soap operas to target specific social problems, including the prevention of blindness. What are needed are programmes that interest people without trying to force a message on them. We believe that with the growth of television and improvement in its programming we will be able to achieve substantial gains in the level of health of our people.

Blindness, especially in a country as culturally and economically diverse as India, cannot be tackled by proclaiming fiats from Delhi or other high-level directives. Problems must be solved through the involvement of people at all levels. Prevention of blindness programmes must be able to differentiate specific problems. Such programmes must be decentralized so that they can be tailored to the specific zones and particular people for whom they are targeted. For them to be successful we have to see that the normal bureaucratic red tape does not tie them up or even slow them down. Of course, with modern technology all the red tape is much stronger and it has become much harder to cut through. But this is something we are committed to do in our prevention of blindness programme and we have the people to carry it out.

For this programme to be most effective we must involve the people at the grassroots level—not just the doctors, surgeons, and medical assistants, but the local people as well. To accomplish this we have brought the Health Ministry and the Human Resources Development Ministry together to attack the problems of preventing blindness. What we are looking for is more than just improving health, because sometimes we cannot improve health to the degree we would like. What we want to do is to give every human being as complete a life as possible—whatever his particular problems and hardships may be. By bringing these two ministries together we hope to make them more helpful to the people we are trying to reach.

Finally, let me thank you for coming to Delhi and honouring us with your Third General Assembly and for helping us stimulate the prevention of blindness programme in India. I have no doubt that your deliberations, both those in which you will sketch out broad programmes and those in which you will work out minute details, will give a significant impetus to blindness prevention. Let me wish you all the best in your work. We look forward to working with you to remove blindness from India and from the rest of the world.

3

A decade of progress in the prevention of blindness

Carl Kupfer
President, IAPB

In considering blindness and efforts to prevent it, we can choose between two radically different perspectives. One is a very sombre picture. It shows more than 40 million people blind and untold millions with lesser degrees of visual impairment. Onchocerciasis, cataract, xerophthalmia, glaucoma, and other diseases continue to claim the sight of millions every year.

Furthermore, on the horizon is the threat of an increase in blindness because of demographic changes: as populations grow larger and their median age rises, more and more people move into the ge brackets in which cataract, glaucoma, and other age-related diseases tend to strike. For example, it has been estimated that in the United States the frequency of cataract will increase by 160 per cent in the next few decades unless preventive measures are found. In the developing world, the population aged 55 and over will increase almost five-fold by the year 2030, with a concomitant increase in all the blinding conditions related to age. In fact, despite all our efforts, some argue that the number of blind people is increasing rather than decreasing.

This grim picture is one that we all carry in our minds as we go about our efforts to combat blindness. And it is necessary that we do this, because it imparts a sense of urgency and realism that is essential to our work.

But we must not forget that there is another perspective—an optimistic side to the prevention of blindness situation. It is this view that I want to concentrate on.

The fact is that the past decade has been a time of extraordinary progress in programmes for the prevention of blindness. We have enormous successes to our credit now, so many that it takes a General Assembly, with speakers and participants drawn from around the globe, to give us a full view of the advances that have occurred. If we reflect upon these hopeful trends and identify the strengths that made them possible, I think we will be well prepared to face the challenges of the future.

The first element of progress that I would point to is the growth in resources for the prevention of blindness over the past decade. And of course the starting point for any such discussion must be the World Health Organization (WHO), because it is paramount. It has been the fountainhead of public health expertise and leadership for much of the world, and has provided technical assistance for the development of a national programme in virtually every country represented here.

Therefore, it is particularly heartening to see how much the WHO Prevention of Blindness Programme has grown. In 1978, when it began, it had just one professional on its staff, and he was based in Geneva. It had no separate budget. In 1980, when the programme was first assigned funds of its own, it had US$1.3 million for two years of operations; and the staff had increased only slightly: there were now two professionals, both in Geneva. But just a few years later, in 1984 and 1985, the picture had changed considerably: the budget had almost doubled to US$2.3 million, and full-time offices had been established in both the South-East Asia region and the region of the Americas.

In addition to the funds allocated to it by WHO, the Prevention of Blindness Programme has attracted extra-budgetary funds from a variety of sources. These include the Japan Shipbuilding Industry Foundation, the Arab Gulf Fund for the United Nations Development Organization (also known as AGFUND), and the United Nations Development Programme. Contributions from these and other donors have provided the WHO Programme with US$7.5 million in extra-budgetary funds over the past five years. Thus WHO is in a position to pursue more prevention of blindness activities now than at any time in the past.

There has been a parallel growth in the resources of the non-governmental organizations that are such an important part of blindness prevention and of the IAPB. For example, in 1975 the Royal Commonwealth Society for the Blind had an annual budget of £424 000 to support all of its overseas activities, and in that year it was able to finance 82 000 cataract operations. But by 1985 the annual overseas budget had risen to £2.8 million, and the society was able to support 249 000 cataract operations. For the decade, the Society has expended £13.8 million overseas. It has financed 2 million cataract surgeries and a total of 20 million eye treatments of various kinds. This is an extraordinary total, and it shows how determination and skill in mobilizing resources can yield a programme that makes a real difference in the lives of many people.

Over the past decade, other non-governmental organizations have experienced a similar growth in resources. These include Helen Keller International, the Christoffel-Blindenmission, the International Eye Foundation, Operation Eyesight Universal, and the Seva Foundation. The five organizations I just mentioned, together with Royal Commonwealth Society for the Blind, expended more than US$30 million on blindness prevention and related activities in 1985. The comparable figure for 1975 was only US$6 million.

This growth means that these organizations now command the resources to support sizeable programmes that have a highly noticeable impact. The cataract surgery programmes sponsored by Royal Commonwealth Society for the Blind, Christoffel-Blindenmission, Operation Eyesight Universal, and the Seva Foundation are one example. The massive vitamin A supplementation programmes begun by Helen Keller International are another. The programmes for training allied health personnel sponsored by the International Eye Foundation are a third. There is every reason to believe that the growth in resources that makes such programmes possible will continue in the future.

In view of this increase in resources and expansion of programmes, it is very fortunate that we have achieved excellent co-ordination between WHO and the non-governmental organizations concerned with the prevention of blindness.

Through the IAPB, the non-governmental organizations regularly consult with WHO. We meet every other year. In the alternate years, the policy advisory group for the WHO Prevention of Blindness Programme meets to exchange ideas and make suggestions about WHO plans and activities. Also, the non-governmental organizations hold partnership meetings to co-ordinate their activities. These meetings, along with frequent informal contacts throughout the year, keep the international effort against blindness one of the best co-ordinated among all health programmes.

Our perception of the importance of co-ordinating prevention of blindness activities was heightened at the World Health Congress in Geneva in 1985. At that meeting the major technical discussions centred on the need for increased collaboration between the WHO and non-governmental organizations. The IAPB exhibit and presentation drew considerable attention from the delegates. That was because we demonstrated how well individual organizations and WHO interact in designing and operating prevention of blindness programmes in Latin America, Asia, and Africa.

Communications have been further enhanced by the *IAPB News*. This very valuable medium summarizes recent prevention of blindness accomplishments and newly initiated programmes around the world. Activities of WHO, the non-governmental organizations, and—most important—the national committees are highlighted in the *IAPB News*. Several years ago, this newsletter was published annually, and only a few hundred copies were printed. Now it is produced twice-yearly and its circulation has grown to include more than 2300 people in 135 countries. Through it, each reader can keep abreast of prevention of blindness activities around the world. Also, the newsletter provides each group with an opportunity to tell a world-wide audience about its activities and thereby generate widespread interest.

We can see an increase in strength and co-ordination at the national level also. Governments are increasingly recognizing the importance of blindness prevention activities. A decade ago, very few governments saw the necessity for a national plan to prevent blindness. But today, almost 60 countries have national plans for the prevention of blindness, and at least 45 of those have fully-fledged programmes. This interest on the part of governments reflects a growing awareness of the fact that prevention of blindness programmes have several desirable features: they yield highly visible short-term results and require only modest additional resources. Also, money for their support is often available from international sources, and they can be fitted within the health infrastructure that the country already possesses.

Another factor accounting for this upsurge in activity at the national level is the growth in influence of the national committees that act as a focus for prevention of blindness activities within their respective countries. National committees play an important role in influencing governments to turn to WHO for help in designing prevention of blindness programmes. Also, the IAPB committees are instrumental in raising funds, in working with voluntary organizations such as the Lions and Rotary Clubs, and in co-operating with international non-governmental organizations and WHO country representatives to develop prevention of blindness programmes.

We have an excellent example of a well-constituted and highly active national committee in India. It contains individuals with a wealth of public health experience, political adeptness, and technological know-how, and it is interacting closely with the government's Ministry of Health. This is just the sort of interaction that is essential in the sequence of events leading to an effective programme: first, there must be an increase in commitment at the national level. With the help of WHO, this commitment is then expressed by the development of a national plan. The plan can be used as the basis for attracting resources, and these make it possible to implement the plan through co-operation between the government and the non-governmental organizations. This sequence of events has now taken place in scores of countries, resulting in the initiation of prevention of blindness programmes in many areas that were without eye care a decade ago.

Another trend which is of great importance is one that was emphasized at our last General Assembly. Those who attended will undoubtedly recall that Dr Robert Muller, Assistant Secretary-General of the United Nations, spoke to us about the need to base our programmes on firm data about the causes, prevalence, and distribution of blindness. Within the last few years there has been a surge of activity to achieve this. There have been major surveys in Indonesia, China, Saudi Arabia, Nepal, and in several African countries.

Information from these surveys is being used well. The studies have been closely linked to intervention efforts, and thus are contributing to the design of well-targeted and cost-effective programmes which rest on a base of knowledge that was not available to us 10 years ago, or even a few years ago.

Another encouraging trend of the past decade is that prevention of blindness programmes have become increasingly innovative. We are continually finding new forms of intervention that are low in cost, safe, and highly effective.

As an example, I would point to the evolution of the programmes to prevent xerophthalmia by increasing vitamin A intake. Initially, all these programmes were based on supplementation by means of vitamin A in capsules or solution. This remains a feature of most of these programmes. But new approaches have also emerged. One of these is fortification, which makes it possible to achieve rapid and widespread distribution of vitamin A. Another new strategy, which may be even more promising in the long run, is the educational approach that teaches mothers to use naturally occurring sources of vitamin A from the local environment in the family diet. Where education succeeds, people will be safe from vitamin A deficiency for generations. That is an enormous impact, and it can be realized through a programme that in the long run is relatively low in cost.

Ongoing innovation is also evident in the ophthalmic outreach programmes that have evolved here in India and elsewhere. Eye camps and mobile eye units were striking new concepts when they originated several decades ago, and over the past decade they have continued to demonstrate that it is possible to deliver safe cataract surgery for just a few dollars per patient. Now there is increasing emphasis on the rural 'satellite' hospital as a fixed peripheral facility for ophthalmic care. Improving patients' access to such centres, as well as improving access to the base hospital, is one of the major challenges we now face. In the meantime, the eye camps and mobile units continue to be of great importance. A renewed effort is being made to improve both safety and efficiency, so that even more patients can be treated.

Other highly innovative activities are the ophthalmic training programmes now being conducted in Thailand, Bangladesh, and the Caribbean. In these programmes, general practitioners are being taught to perform cataract surgery. These low-cost programmes to expand the pool of trained ophthalmic manpower have significantly increased the number of sight-restoring operations performed each year.

These programmes also illustrate how much our awareness of the problem of cataract has increased over the past decade. Ten years ago, we were alert to the dangers posed by infectious diseases such as trachoma and onchocerciasis, but we were less aware of cataract as a cause of avoidable blindness. Now, as a result of surveys and careful re-examination of our patient population, we can see how high this disease ranks as a cause of blindness. In fact, we now know that cataract is the major cause of avoidable blindness in almost all regions of the developing world. And we can adjust our priorities accordingly. This need to set priorities was one of the challenges I emphasized at the last General Assembly, and I am very pleased to see how far we have progressed in this regard in just four years.

Another very encouraging trend is that science and technology are continuing to give us new and better tools suitable for large-scale programmes to combat blindness. We witnessed a massive application of advanced technology in the Upper Volta River Basin Project, which used aircraft and highly effective pesticides to kill the black-fly that carries onchocerciasis. Now the fly has been eradicated in 80 per cent of the programme area. Also, in many villages where onchocerciasis was once rampant, there are no infected children under the age of 10.

However, around the world there are still 28 million people who have onchocerciasis. For them, scientific research has yielded a promising new drug called Ivermectin, which appears to be safe and effective for use on a mass scale. Ivermectin may offer a means of medically controlling onchocerciasis, even in residual areas that are still infested by the black-fly.

Other highly useful technological advances that have been made available at low cost include the portable cryoprobe for cataract surgery. And soon we may also have the portable YAG laser being developed for performing both therapeutic and prophylactic irido-tomies in people with narrow-angle glaucoma. This increasing access to new and appropriate technology will strengthen our ability to deliver safe and cost-effective treatments on a mass scale.

Also, because of all the advances I have mentioned and our new knowledge about the causes and distribution of blindness, we are better equipped than ever to demonstrate the value of programmes for the prevention of blindness. We can prove the reduction in prevalence and the concomitant cost-effectiveness of these efforts. This gives us an even better chance of attracting the resources needed to support large-scale programmes to combat blindness.

In summary, the IAPB and its member groups have long had the determination to be highly effective. Now we have the resources, the organization, and the knowledge to accomplish more than ever before. Seen from this perspective, the past decade has been one of astounding success—probably greater success than any of us would have predicted 10 years ago.

In the future, we must maintain our momentum. It is essential that we continue to make well-designed plans, marshal resources, and initiate and maintain effective programmes. We must do this because we face a formidable challenge, not only from blinding diseases, but also from the potential increase in blindness associated with the rising age of populations.

But set against this challenge is the increasing effectiveness of this organization, and the steadfast faith we all share: that we can make a difference and that we can continue to mount programmes eminently worthy of support. By drawing on the strengths and experiences that have brought us to this point, we will succeed in advancing the world-wide campaign against avoidable blindness.

4

Four main causes of blindness

TRACHOMA

Bjorn Thylefors and Chandler R. Dawson

Definition

Trachoma is a highly contagious eye disease that affects about 360 million people world-wide. Approximately 6 to 9 million are blind from trachoma and an estimated 80 million children are in need of treatment. The disease is most common in the drier regions of the developing countries. It is particularly frequent in northern and subsaharan Africa, the Middle East, and parts of South-East Asia.

Trachoma is associated with poverty, overcrowding, lack of clean water and personal hygiene, and poor sanitation. Under suitable conditions, the disease spreads rapidly.

Early signs of trachoma include reddening, burning, and watering of the eyes. These signs are caused by inflammation of the conjunctiva, and without treatment may subside spontaneously or progress to scarring. It also causes the cornea to become inflamed with the growth of blood vessels over it. The most serious corneal damage, however, occurs when the scarred conjunctiva contracts and causes the eyelids to become inverted, so that the eyelashes rub against the cornea (trichiasis). This constant, painful abrasion can cause corneal ulcers, perforations, and scarring that may result in blindness.

Although infection with the trachoma-causing organism (*Chlamydia trachomatis*) usually occurs in childhood, visual loss most often happens during adult years. In general, blindness does not result until 10 to 20 years after the initial infection.

Trachoma can be treated effectively with topically administered antibiotics and other drugs. However, unless behavioural and environmental factors that favour the spread of the disease are corrected, the infection may recur. The importance of personal hygiene, particularly face-washing amongst children, has been demonstrated as one example of behavioural aspects of trachoma control which must be addressed in health education. Surgical correction of inturned eyelids is an effective method to prevent corneal opacities and visual loss.

Progress

Trachoma has been eliminated already from the most developed regions of the world through the improvement in living conditions that has accompanied industrialization. In other areas where trachoma remains endemic, community-wide control programmes based on the mass application of topical antibiotics, accompanied by environmental health measures, have been found effective in reducing the frequency and severity of the disease. Surgical correction of in-turned eyelids is an integral part of blindness prevention, and has often been carried out by non-specialist health workers with special training. There are ongoing effective trachoma control programmes, often forming part of primary eye care, in several countries, such as Botswana, Brazil, Burma, Fiji, Oman, Sudan, Tunisia, and Vietnam. In many other developing countries, trachoma has been brought under control as a cause of blindness, even though the disease is still endemic in certain parts of those countries. Nonetheless, the continuing toll of visual loss from trachoma amongst many populations in developing countries indicates a need for continued extensive efforts to combat this disease.

Strategy

1. Systematic assessment programmes should be used to identify communities where blinding trachoma is endemic.
2. High priority should be assigned to detecting trachoma and reducing its prevalence amongst young children.
3. Mass treatment with topical tetracycline should be undertaken in any community where the prevalence of trachoma amongst children is 20 per cent or more.
4. Adults should be included along with children in trachoma screening programmes.
5. Screening should be designed to identify cases of trichiasis and entropion (the sight-threatening eyelid deformities caused by trachoma) requiring surgery. The effectiveness of this surgery should be assessed.
6. Attention should be given to non-medical measures that can reduce the incidence of trachoma. These include economic development and improvement of water supplies and sanitation.

XEROPHTHALMIA

Barbara A. Underwood

Problem definition

Xerophthalmia blinds annually an estimated 250 000 children in Asia alone and temporarily or permanently impairs the vision of millions more. Recent surveys conducted in African countries are uncovering areas where xerophthalmia at a level of public health significance was not previously recognized, and in some Latin American countries there is growing evidence of pockets of populations at high risk of clinical disease. There is little doubt, therefore, that the estimate for nutrition-related blindness in Asia vastly underestimates the global problem for which accurate estimates are unavailable. Tragically, in addition to its blinding consequences, severe xerophthalmia is associated with a high mortality rate. Recent evidence suggests that the mortality toll is even greater than previously suspected because depletion in vitamin A also increases the risk of lethal infections among those who are only mildly or subclinically affected.

Xerophthalmia is the result of prolonged vitamin A deficiency and in its irreversible blinding manifestation (keratomalacia) is most often associated with a preceding acute systemic or enteric infectious episode such as measles, diarrhoea, or respiratory infections, or with concurrent severe protein-calorie deficiency. It may also occur secondary to prolonged malabsorption syndromes. The blinding form of xerophthalmia primarily afflicts the youngest age groups and is most often associated with impoverished circumstances, malnutrition, and infections. Milder forms are more frequent in males. Milder manifestations of xerophthalmia (nightblindness) are sometimes reported among pregnant and lactating women.

The term xerophthalmia describes a series of symptoms and signs of progressively increasing severity that affect the retina, conjunctiva, and cornea. The earliest symptom is nightblindness caused by an inadequate regeneration of rhodopsin in the retina after exposure to bright light. This symptom, which is readily reversible, causes young children to stumble when they go from outside play into a darkened room or young women to complain of poor vision when they enter their house after working in the fields. Conjunctival xerosis (dryness) follows and is often associated with the appearance of Bitot spots, a heaping up of desquamated epithelial cells usually on the temporal side of the conjunctiva. Bitot spots may be unilateral or bilateral and sometimes occur nasally. Among preschool-aged children they are nearly always indicative of current vitamin A deficiency and are readily responsive to vitamin A therapy, but among older children and adults Bitot spots may reflect past vitamin A inadequacy and be slower to respond to vitamin A therapy. In the absence of vitamin A therapy, the cornea is affected next, developing a punctate keratopathy, which is observable with a portable slit lamp, as well as dryness and cloudiness. These symptoms also are quickly reversible upon treatment with vitamin A. If untreated, however, rapid progression may occur in which the cornea softens, ulcerates, and may perforate with irreversible partial or complete blindness. Rapid therapy with vitamin A may at least partially save vision if given prior to perforation. Treatment schedules call for high doses of vitamin A provided orally (200 000 iu immediately upon diagnosis and again the following day) or intramuscular injections of water-miscible (100 000 iu immediately and the oral dose the following day) when diarrhoea or severe vomiting are associated problems.

As a public health concern, blindness from vitamin A deficiency (xerophthalmia/keratomalacia) is a social not a medical problem. It is the result of habitually eating too little of foods with vitamin A activity. This may be for economic, social, or cultural reasons. Foods that contain vitamin A in its natural preformed form are relatively expensive (animal protein products such as eggs, whole milk, liver) and infrequently eaten by those at highest risk of clinical deficiency (preschool-aged children). Foods that contain the less expensive precursor form (carotenoid-containing such as yellow fruits and vegetables and dark green leafy vegetables) are either very seasonal (mango, papaya, buriti) or for social/cultural reasons considered not to be suitable food for humans or for feeding young children (drumstick leaves, amaranth, spinach).

Progress

Xerophthalmia, as noted above, is largely a social problem and it has disappeared from previously endemic areas as economic and/or social changes have bought about improvements in health, nutrition, and the standard of living. In some instances, where clinical deficiency was not an acute public health concern, no specific programme to provide high-dose supplements was required; social and economic redistribution of resources (for example, China) or enhancement (for example, Costa Rica) was sufficient. In areas where the occurrence is at a level to require public health attention, high-dose vitamin supplements have been needed to relieve the acute situation and provide for a transition to the period when other long-term measures become effective (for example, Indonesia). In the last decade, among some countries progress has occurred in going from less efficient universal distribution of high-dose supplements on a six-monthly basis to distribution through programmes targeted to high-risk groups (for example, Haiti). Consideration is now being given to incorporating the high-dose supplementation into the schedule for immunization programmes and into programmes for treatment and follow-up of diarrhoeal disease and measles. In all endemic areas, the high-dose supplement remains an essential element for treatment that should be available in health facilities.

Food fortification with vitamin A has contributed significantly to maintaining an adequate level of vitamin A nutrition in industrialized countries. Potentially it is a strategy appropriate for use in non-industrialized areas, where intakes of vitamin A by the general population are low. Progress in implementing fortification programmes in these areas, however, has had variable success. These programmes are technically feasible where an appropriate dietary vehicle can be identified, but implementation has been impeded by political and economic problems. The sugar fortification programme in Guatemala, for example, although demonstrated to be successful technically and in improving the population's intake level of vitamin A, was stopped for other reasons and negotiations still have not been successful in reinstituting the programme. In other countries, such as Indonesia and the Philippines, widespread fortification programmes, although technically ready for implementation, have not received full national political backing. In Bangladesh and India the prevention programmes continue to rely upon high-dose distribution in capsule or liquid form. No suitable fortification vehicle has been identified.

Increasingly, efforts are being made to involve communities in solving their own problem of an inadequate intake of vitamin A. Efforts are being made to stimulate the production of vitamin A-rich foods in home gardens and in helping mothers to know how to use these effectively in child diets.

Health and nutrition education is being incorporated into innovative communication programmes and social marketing techniques are being applied to expand the population outreach. These programmes focus on improved knowledge of available vitamin A-rich foods suitable for child diets and couple this information with health and nutrition education programmes to improve consumption and dietary patterns and to reduce environmental health hazards.

ONCHOCERCIASIS

Hugh R. Taylor

Definition

Onchocerciasis is the blinding human disease caused by infection with the filarial worm *Onchocerca volvulus*. It affects some 28 million people in Africa and Latin America. It is transmitted by small, biting black-flies that breed in rapids along the rivers of large areas of West and Central Africa and in smaller areas of Latin and South America. In areas in which it is endemic, onchocerciasis has a devastating impact. Almost everyone will be infected by adolescence, most will have some degree of the debilitating skin changes, two out of five people will become blind, and those that are blind have one-third the life expectancy of the sighted.[1] Particularly in West Africa, villages of subsistance farmers along the fertile rivers are decimated and ultimately abandoned.

Until now there has not been a satisfactory way of treating onchocerciasis. For the past 60 years, two drugs have been in limited use for treating onchocerciasis—diethylcarbamazine (DEC) and Suramin. Both drugs cause dangerous and at times life-threatening side-effects, and their use has been generally restricted to only those with the most severe sight-threatening disease and only then under close medical supervision.[2] For that reason, there has been essentially no way to reach the millions of people who continue to suffer from onchocerciasis or the 1 to 2 million people who have become blind.

An ambitious, large, long-term control programme has operated in the worst affected areas of West Africa for the last decade. This programme, the Onchocerciasis Control Programme (OCP), was established by the World Health Organization (WHO), the World Bank, and other United Nations agencies. The OCP has aimed at stopping the transmission of onchocerciasis by eliminating the black-fly vectors.[3] It has done that by spraying the breeding sites of the black-fly with a selective larvicide. This has been no mean task as the breeding sites are often relatively inaccessible. Also, they must be sprayed by air—usually by helicopter—and constantly change as the water flow changes during the rainy and dry seasons. Despite many difficulties, it has been outstandingly effective and has essentially eliminated the transmission of infection in an area of over 700 000 square kilometres involving seven countries. It is now planned to extend this programme and almost double the area it covers and include portions of four more countries.

The OCP has provided a protective umbrella for about one-quarter of those with onchocerciasis. But because of logistic and economic reasons, similar programmes in other areas of onchocerciasis are not feasible, so the future for those living in these areas looks bleak.

Progress

Recently, however, there has been a major advance in the prospects for a safe and effective drug that can be used on a large scale to treat onchocerciasis. Ivermectin is a new drug which has been evaluated recently in patients infected with onchocerciasis.[4,5,6] These studies suggest that Ivermectin is not only extremely effective in reducing the level of infection but that it is also much safer than the previously available drugs for treating onchocerciasis.

In man, the onchocerciasis parasite develops into male and female adult worms that reproduce sexually and the female worm releases millions of tiny worms or microfilariae. The microfilariae migrate throughout the body but especially to the skin and the eye. Much of the pathology that is seen in onchocerciasis is thought to be due to the severe reaction that forms around dead microfilariae. Drugs such as DEC kill microfilariae and cause a severe reaction known as the Mazzotti reaction which can lead to visual loss and seriously limits the usefulness of such drugs. Ivermectin is at least as effective as DEC in reducing the levels of microfilariae in the skin and the eye[6,7] but without the severe reaction.[8] So far, the mechanism of action of Ivermectin against the microfilariae is unknown although its main pharmacological effect is that of a gabba agonist.

Ivermectin does not kill the adult worms of *O. volvulus*, so a single course of Ivermectin is not curative. It does, however, appear to have some effect on the uterus of the female worm so that the rate at which microfilariae can repopulate the skin and eye after Ivermectin treatment is much slower than after DEC. A further benefit of Ivermectin treatment is a reduction in the uptake of microfilariae by black-flies[9] that suggests that Ivermectin treatment could also significantly reduce transmission.

The most striking thing about Ivermectin is that these

outstanding results have followed a tiny single oral dose. Mass distribution programmes will probably use an annual single oral dose of only 150 μg/kg of Ivermectin possibly given just before the start of the transmission season. Such a programme could be based within the context of a country's primary health care programme. It should not only offer optimal treatment to those already infected but also provide protection to others by reducing transmission. Large community-based studies are now planned in several countries to test the safety and efficacy of Ivermectin given as a mass treatment.

Strategy

Only one paper was presented on onchocerciasis, but it reported the first results of repeated treatment with Ivermectin.[10] However, the following strategies have been given priority by the World Health Organization.[11]

1. *Chemotherapy*
   (a) to develop new filaricides, especially macrofilaricides; and
   (b) to improve the use of currently available drugs.

2. *Immunology and pathology*
   (a) to improve immunodiagnostic techniques especially by the detection of parasite antigens;
   (b) to determine the mechanisms of both natural and treatment-induced immunopathology and identify predictive factors;
   (c) to develop better animal models; and
   (d) to assess the possibility of protection by vaccination.

3. *Field research*
   (a) to identify risk factors for disease;
   (b) to improve methods of identifying parasites in vectors; and
   (c) to improve methods of controlling vectors.

References

1. Prost, A. and Vaugelade, J. (1981). La surmortalite des aveugles en zone de Savane Ouest-Africaine. *Bulletin of the World Health Organization (Geneva)*, **59**, 773–6.
2. Taylor, H.R. (1984). Recent developments in the treatment of onchocerciasis. *Bulletin of the World Health Organization (Geneva)*, **62**, 509–15.
3. Bland, J. (1985). A decade of oncho control. *World Health (Geneva)*, October, 1–27.

4. Awadzi, K., Dadzie, K.Y., Schulz-Key, H., Haddock, D.R.W., Gilles, H.M., and Aziz, M.A. (1985). The chemotherapy of onchocerciasis X. An assessment of four single-dose treatment regimes of M K-933 (ivermectin) in human onchocerciasis. *Annals of Tropical Medicine and Parasitology (London)*, **79**, 63–78.

5. Aziz, M.A., Diallo, S., Diop, I.M., and Lariviere, M. (1982). Efficacy and tolerance of ivermectin in human onchocerciasis. *Lancet (London)*, **2**, 171–3.

6. Greene, B.M. *et al.* (1985). Comparison of Ivermectin and diethylcarbamazine in the treatment of onchocerciasis. *New England Journal of Medicine (Boston)*, **313**, 133–8.

7. Larivierre, M. *et. al.* (1985). Double-blind study of Ivermectin and diethylcarbamazine in African onchocerciasis patients with ocular involvement. *Lancet (London)*, **2**, 174–7.

8. Taylor, H.R. *et al.* (1986). Comparison of the treatment of ocular onchocerciasis with ivermectin and diethylcarbamazine. *Archives of Ophthalmology (Chicago)*, **104**, 863–70.

9. Cupp, E.W. *et al.* (1986). The effects of Ivermectin on transmission of *Onchocerca volvulus*. *Science (Washington)*, **231**, 740–2.

10. Newland, H.S., White, A.T., Greene, B.M., and Taylor, H.R. (1986). *The effect of repeated treatment with Ivermectin in onchocerciasis*. Paper presented at Third General Assembly of International Agency for the Prevention of Blindness, New Delhi, India.

11. Scientific Working Group on Filariasis, Geneva. *Workplan for filariasis*. Geneva UNDP/World Bank/WHO Special Programme for Research and Training in Tropical Diseases, January 1986.

CATARACT

Carl Kupfer

Definition and overview

A cataract is an opacity in the lens that interferes with vision. If it reduces visual acuity to 20/30 (6/9) or less, a visual disability is said to exist. However, the international definition of blindness due to cataract is the inability to count fingers at a distance of 3 metres. Using this definition of blindness, there are 14 to 17 million cataract blind, a major proportion of which could probably have sight restored by cataract surgery.

It is now generally recognized that, throughout the developing world, cataract is the main cause of blindness, accounting for at least one-half of all blindness. Of particular importance is that blindness caused by cataract is curable at a reasonably low cost from the Western point of view of about US$25 for each patient.

Because this problem in the developing world involves a huge backlog of unoperated cataract patients, plus the new cases that develop every year, it is of staggering economic proportions. The cost of treatment already represents a major expenditure in public health funds, and the situation is rapidly worsening as the population ages and the demand for cataract surgery increases.

The major impediments to the delivery of adequate cataract services in the developing world are the scarcity of trained manpower, the lack of facilities—especially in rural areas, the social and economic barriers to cataract surgery that prevent individuals from coming forward for treatment, and the overall increase in the number of cataract blind because of the growing number of the elderly in the population.

Strategy

There are three broad approaches to reducing the prevalence of cataract. Two approaches are long-term: using epidemiology to determine the risk factors in cataract and understanding the molecular biology of cataract formation so that medical means to slow down or prevent cataract formation can be developed. It should be noted that if cataract formation could be delayed by 10 years, the number of individuals needing cataract surgery would be reduced by 45 per cent. The third approach, which is short-term, is addressing the problem of those individuals already blind from cataract. This includes using operations research methodology to determine the optimal approach to each of the aspects of the delivery of cataract services. These would include assessment of the problem in each locale, creation of awareness of the problem of cataract in the population, case finding at the community level, development of a referral system, motivation to help the cataract blind use this system to be examined and undergo surgery, provision of low-cost but high-quality surgical services for treating a large number of patients, and provision of low-cost optical correction. To the extent possible, case finding and referral should be carried out at the primary health care level. Visual acuity measurement and identification of a white pupil can be incorporated into the training of community health workers. Referral for further examination and surgery, if necessary, should be to more qualified individuals competent to determine the need for surgery and to perform a safe and successful operation. A team approach in the management of the facilities and conduct of the surgical procedure will increase the capacity of the system without sacrificing safety.

An example of an effort to reduce the backlog of the cataract blind in a well-defined urban area is provided in Appendix D. Finally, the report—including specific recommendations—of a WHO Inter-regional Meeting on the Management of Cataract within Primary Health Care Systems is included in Appendix E.

5

Regional action

AFRICA

The World Health Organization (WHO) Programme for the Prevention of Blindness was established in the African Region in 1978. On
the basis of surveys and publications from several parts of Africa,
blindness has been found to be a public health problem of major
importance. These surveys have also indicated that the highest
blindness prevalence rates in the world are to be found in some
African countries. The commonest causes of blindness in Africa are
onchocerciasis, trachoma, cataract, vitamin A deficiency, measles,
and trauma. Endeavours to prevent the emergence of blindness
have been hampered by the lack of awareness of the risk factors and
the paucity of human and material resources. When available, these
resources are mainly confined to urban centres and are mostly in the
form of curative and restorative services, with none at all made
available in rural areas, where a majority of people live.

There is a general lack of information regarding causes and frequency of blindness in this region. WHO has therefore collaborated
with member states and several non-governmental organizations in
carrying out blindness surveys. In addition, WHO is participating
in the training of ophthalmic medical auxiliaries at the Lilongwe
Auxiliary Training Institute in Malawi. Several other African
countries have instituted personnel training programmes. The African Institute of Tropical Ophthalmology (IOTA), based at Bamako,
Mali, has been redesignated as a WHO Collaborating Centre and is
engaged in training as well as research.

In September 1980, 23 participants attended a subregional
workshop on prevention of blindness in Lilongwe. This was followed
by another seminar held in Accra, Ghana, in 1982, which was
attended by 15 participants. In 1983, Zambia organized a national
symposium in collaboration with WHO. In April of the following
year, representatives attended a subregional seminar on prevention
of blindness in Kampala, Uganda. Also in 1984, 74 participants
representing 12 countries and several non-governmental organizations met at a scientific meeting on blindness prevention in Moshi,
United Republic of Tanzania. A task force on prevention of blindness

was held in Brazzaville from 20 to 22 October 1986. At that meeting, which was organized by WHO, representatives of several member states, non-governmental organizations, and UNICEF reviewed the blindness situation in Africa and made recommendations relating to suitable strategies for its prevention, including resource mobilization.

In 1986 WHO procured drugs and equipment worth US$20 000 for both Chad and Uganda. The blindness prevention programme also participated in a survey being carried out on the schoolchildren of Ouagadougou, Burkina Faso, and contributed towards the organization of a national seminar on blindness held in Mauritania during December.

Ten African nations are participating in the Onchocerciasis Control Programme sponsored by the United Nations Development Programme (UNDP), the Food and Agriculture Organization (FAO), and the World Bank. WHO acts as executive agency for this programme, which has succeeded in eliminating the black-fly from 90 per cent of the programme area. During an examination of over 6000 children born since commencement of operations in the nations of Benin, Burkina Faso, Ghana, the Ivory Coast, Mali, and Niger, only one child has contracted onchocerciasis. This is dramatic evidence of the success of this programme, which will be extended to Guinea, Guinea-Bissau, Senegal, and Sierra Leone.

Other regional activities include the one being conducted by Helen Keller International (HKI) in the Sahel region. The participating nations are Burkina Faso, Chad, Mali, and Niger. Three teams have been assembled to perform assessments of nutritional blindness and trachoma among young children in this region. Following evaluation of these assessments, HKI plans to implement a programme for the prevention of blindness in these areas.

Also, the Christoffel-Blindenmission (CBM) has an extensive prevention of blindness programme in Africa. In collaboration with local churches and mission societies, CBM supports 159 medical projects in 39 countries. Ophthalmic and preventive care is given to the blind, the visually handicapped, and the sick through eye hospitals, community health centres, mobile eye services, dispensaries, and eye departments of general hospitals.

The Royal Commonwealth Society for the Blind (RCSB) is also active in Africa, supporting activities that include Sight by Wings safaris, a training course for ophthalmic paramedical workers, and training awards for students. Another regional programme is the Southern African Sub-regional Ophthalmic Training Centre at the Lilongwe School for Health Sciences in Malawi. The school is sponsored by RCSB, Operation Eyesight Universal (OEU), CBM, and WHO.

Through WHO, the Japan Shipbuilding Industry Foundation has also contributed to the support of prevention of blindness programmes in Africa. Other activities in specific countries are summarized as follows:

Burkina Faso   The headquarters for the WHO Onchocerciasis Control Programme are at Ouagadougou in Burkina Faso. Other activities here include those of OEU which supports ophthalmic nurses in the north-western region of the country.

Ethiopia   When high rates of xerophthalmia were discovered among children during the recent famine in this region, HKI began a programme to provide vitamin A for the treatment and prevention of nutritional blindness. The programme trained health workers and shipped 2 million vitamin A capsules to Ethiopia for distribution. Although emergency xerophthalmia has diminished, HKI continues to provide assistance to those who are at risk of nutritional blindness because of chronic malnutrition.

The International Eye Foundation (IEF) is also active in Ethiopia. To aid in the establishment of an effective eye care system, IEF plans to assist the Government in the development of secondary-level ophthalmic manpower. In collaboration with HKI, the Ministry of Health, and the faculty of medicine at Addis Ababa University, IEF will establish a one-year training programme to provide primary eye care workers for unserved rural areas.

Gambia   With support from the National Eye Institute of the United States, WHO conducted a major survey of blindness and eye disease in the Gambia.

Kenya   IEF's Kenya Rural Blindness Prevention Project was completed in 1984. Through this project, several hundred health workers received training in primary eye care and blindness prevention. This training enabled them to provide essential services in areas without regular eye care. IEF has continued to supervise the Primary Eye Care and Blindness Prevention Education Unit of the Ministry of Health. From 1984 through 1985, over 2000 health workers and primary school teachers received training through this unit.

RCSB also supports the eye care education unit of the Ministry of Health. In addition, RCSB contributes to the support of 19 mobile eye units and a full-time ophthalmologist, and provides ophthalmic equipment for clinical officers.

OEU supports 11 mobile eye units in Kenya and supplies them with needed drugs. Also, OEU is financing a programme to train clinical officers in cataract surgery and is contributing to the expansion of hospital eye departments.

Malawi In 1983 the IEF in collaboration with other agencies conducted a major blindness prevalence survey and study of nutritional eye disease in children in the Lower Shire Valley of Malawi. A major programme to reduce childhood mortality and visual loss was launched by the IEF in 1985. Other prevention of blindness activities in Malawi include the training programme at the Lilongwe School, mentioned earlier, and mobile eye units financed by OEU and RCSB.

Mali The French Organization for the Prevention of Blindness (OPC) is supporting the Yeelen Project in Mali and neighbouring countries of French-speaking Africa. The project utilizes regional centres created at hospitals and motorized teams to combat blindness from trachoma, onchocerciasis, and xerophthalmia.

Sudan As in Ethiopia, HKI is providing vitamin A for the treatment and prevention of nutritional blindness. Half a million doses of liquid vitamin A were sent to the Sudan to combat the emergency caused by the famine, and HKI's technical assistance field staff continues to monitor the need for nutritional supplementation and the procedures by which supplies are distributed. Other non-governmental organizations, the United Nations agencies, and industrial corporations are collaborating in this effort.

Tanzania Full funding for the national prevention of blindness plan has been guaranteed by RCSB and CBM. The two organizations already support 13 mobile eye units manned by ophthalmic assistant medical officers. Nurse training and an outreach programme are supported by RCSB at Kilimanjaro Christian Medical Centre. CBM has provided in-service training courses in Malawi for auxiliary eye care workers from 12 African nations. Steps are being taken to integrate eye care services into the primary health care delivery system, particularly in the area of health education.

Also, HKI is working in concert with the National Prevention of Blindness Committee, the Ministry of Health, RCSB, and CBM in a prevention of blindness project in northern Tanzania. The project has developed a system for performing cataract surgery which can be employed in areas where resources are poor, and has also demonstrated a delivery system for the control of trachoma and other infectious diseases. In addition, HKI and Johns Hopkins University are undertaking a major study of trachoma risk factors in central Tanzania.

Zambia RCSB is supporting four mobile eye units in Zambia. With a grant from the US Agency for International Development, HKI has initiated a prevention of blindness project in the Luapala Valley. In close collaboration with the Ministry of Health and the Zambia Flying Doctor Services, HKI has developed an intensive training programme which will graduate 10 to 15 nurses and medical assistants each year and thus improve the quality of eye care.

Zimbabwe With RCSB support, ophthalmic paramedical workers are being trained in Zimbabwe, and an ophthalmic graduate training programme is underway at the University of Munich. RCSB, CBM, and IEF are giving support to rural eye care services, including base hospital units and six mobile eye units. Also, RCSB and IEF are assisting in the reorganization of Zimbabwe eye care services and the development of the national eye care plan.

EASTERN EUROPE

Union of Soviet Socialist Republics Because the health of the Soviet people is of paramount social value, protection of the populace from health risks is one of the most important social tasks of the state. Prevention of blindness is especially important in this country, where qualified ophthalmic aid, prophylaxis treatment of disease and injury, and rehabilitation of the blind are accessible to everybody.

Due to various preventive measures the number of people handicapped by blindness has dropped. The main causes of blindness in the USSR now are diseases of the central visual system, glaucoma, myopia, cataract, vascular damage, injuries, high myopia, and lens pathology.

Ophthalmic aid for the population is being developed by a wide network of out-patient clinics and stationary institutions, including eye hospitals and departments, doctor's consulting rooms in polyclinics, and medico-sanitary units of industrial enterprises. They have set up special All-Union and Republican centres of eye microsurgery, ophthalmotraumatology, ophthalmo-oncology, anti-glaucoma service, and medico-social rehabilitation of the blind.

Dispensaries are the main source of ophthalmic testing and therapy for most people. Their services include treatment of patients with severe eye diseases, such as glaucoma, myopia, pathology of optic nerve, eye injuries, and virtually all of the visually handicapped. Preventive examinations aimed at the early detection of glaucoma are held in many locations.

Much attention is given to child protection. A special system of ophthalmology for children, including a large network of hospitals, ophthalmologists' medical rooms, eye sanatoriums, specialized schools, and preschool establishments have been set up. Education, instruction, and treatment for children with eye diseases is being developed. Regular compulsory ophthalmologic examination of all children is begun at birth; and observation and treatment of children with myopia, strabismus, amblyopia, glaucoma, retinal disease, and other vision problems has been introduced.

In the USSR there is a close relationship between basic scientists and clinical practitioners, thus promoting rapid realization of scientific achievements and improved ophthalmological treatment of the population. A campaign for sight protection employing mass media is also being developed. It should be stressed that all activity to eliminate blindness, and especially to rehabilitate the blind, is being accomplished in conjunction with the Republican Association of the Blind and through the leadership of the All-Russian Association of the Blind.

The Soviet Union has formed a scientifically grounded system of medico-social rehabilitation of the blind, including a complex of medical, psychological, sociological, pedagogical, and labour-professional programmes. This system aims at rehabilitating health and promoting the ability of the blind to work and become socially integrated. Particular attention is paid to the labour-social rehabilitation of the blind. This rehabilitation programme is defined and controlled by physicians at medical institutions and medical-and-labour assessment commissions, where the importance of prevention of blindness is also stressed.

To co-ordinate the various activities relating to the prevention of blindness and the rehabilitation of those already blind, many All-Union and Republican commissions have been formed in the USSR. In addition, the USSR is willing to share its expertise in sight protection and prevention of blindness with other countries, thus providing selfless assistance to help them cope with blindness.

Participation is mostly with socialist countries that are aiming at improving ophthalmological aid for their populations and preventing blindness.

Czechoslovakia   In this country the main causes of blindness are injuries and congenital diseases. There is a state programme to cope with diabetes, and various measures aimed at preventing diabetic retinopathy are being accomplished within its framework. In addition, much attention has been drawn to preventing visual trauma, and consultations promoting the reduction of congenital eye diseases have been organized.

The Association of the Visually Handicapped of Czechoslovakia provides state-supported activities to put an end to blindness and gives important assistance to the blind by helping them arrange their way of life, secure meaningful employment, and acquire necessary technological aids.

German Democratic Republic   The main causes of blindness in this country are primary glaucoma, retinal detachment, and high myopia. Aged pensioners account for 78 per cent of the blind. Perhaps because of the great activity to maintain children's sight, the percentage of the blind under 18 is less than 2 per cent.

The GDR widely provides its population with 1068 ophthalmologists and 2800 stationary beds in specialized eye departments of clinics. Notable ophthalmological activity, especially in cataract, glaucoma, and heterotropia is being developed. (Children with heterotropia—those aged 5 to 10 are 80 per cent of the cases—are being cured surgically.) There are special schools for weak-sighted children and prophylactic medical examinations for all children and teenagers are being made available throughout the nation. Those with glaucoma and diabetic retinopathy are also being treated at numerous locations. To help prevent congenital ocular diseases, officials of the GDR are increasing the number of genetic consultations popularized by the Association of the Blind of GDR.

Hungary   This nation's efforts to prevent and reduce blindness has made notable advances recently. A great deal of attention has been paid to preventing congenital ocular diseases by providing a network of genetic consultations.

LATIN AMERICA

Prevention of Blindness activities in Latin America are marked by close co-operation between the Pan-American Health Organization (PAHO) and non-governmental organizations (NGOs).

In this region, AGFUND (the Arab Gulf Fund for the United Nations Development Organization), has supported a Project for the Prevention of Blindness in the Americas that has had a great impact on activities in nine countries. They are Belize, Bolivia, Ecuador, El Salvador, Guyana, Haiti, Honduras, Nicaragua, and Paraguay. These countries are developing and improving their national eye health programmes with AGFUND support channelled through the World Health Organization (WHO) and PAHO.

Brazil PAHO has established and helped to maintain a WHO Collaborating Centre for the Prevention of Blindness at the Servicio de Oftalmologica Sanitaria, Secretaria de Salud, São Paulo, Brazil. The centre is concentrating on epidemiology of some important causes of blindness. Also, in collaboration with the IAPB, the Pan-American Association of Ophthalmology (PAAO), and Helen Keller International (HKI), PAHO is sponsoring a local project on community attitudes toward cataract surgery. PAHO is also working with the Ministries of Health and NGOs in Brazil and several other Latin American countries in local efforts to eradicate onchocerciasis, trachoma, and leprosy. In addition, PAHO has sponsored a training seminar at São Paulo University for managers of national programmes in eye health.

Costa Rica In Costa Rica, PAHO—in collaboration with the IAPB, PAAO, and HKI—has initiated a study of community attitudes toward cataract surgery.

Ecuador PAHO is working jointly with several NGOs and the Ministry of Health in Ecuador in local efforts to eradicate onchocerciasis. Also, the International Eye Foundation (IEF) is co-operating with the Ministry of Health in the establishment of an eye care programme in which rural physicians and nurses will be trained in primary eye care and rural screening programmes will be developed. Training will be provided not only to Ministry of Health personnel but also to health workers active in private voluntary organizations.

Guatemala PAHO has established a WHO Collaborating Centre

for the Prevention of Blindness at Dr Rodolfo Robles V Eye and Ear Hospital in Guatemala City. The main activities at this Centre are training of personnel in primary eye care, giving support for the provision of eye care at the rural level, and carrying out field research about the causes of blindness. A survey of eye diseases and causes of blindness is underway in the Department of Chimaltenango. Also, PAHO is collaborating with the Ministry of Health in a programme for the eradication of onchocerciasis and xerophthalmia.

Honduras   With the assistance of PAHO, Honduras is now working to develop its national programme in eye health.

Peru   PAHO, in collaboration with IAPB, PAAO, and HKI, is sponsoring a local project on cataract surgery in the community. HKI began working in Peru in 1982, offering support to the Government's eye health programme Centro Oftalmologico Luciano E. Barrere (COLEB). In the area of rehabilitation, HKI has been co-operating with the Ministry of Education. Having completed a prevalence survey to determine the major causes of blindness, HKI has embarked on a very ambitious plan to significantly reduce the incidence of avoidable blindness. The plan involves training a cadre of primary health workers, including general practitioners, in the prevention of eye diseases and in the early detection, treatment, and referral of individuals with these disorders. The programme concentrates on three rural departments representing the jungle, mountain, and Pacific coastal regions of the country. Primary and secondary care is now available in all three target areas, where originally there was an absence of trained professionals. Operation Eyesight Universal is also contributing to this very effective programme.

Venezuela   The Ministry of Health is collaborating with PAHO and several NGOs in an effort to eradicate blindness caused by leprosy.

MIDDLE EAST

Within the past few years, the World Health Organization (WHO) has more than doubled its support for prevention of blindness activities in the Middle East. The main objectives of the WHO Regional Plan for this area are to reduce avoidable blindness to the lowest possible level and to provide essential eye care to under-served populations. Strategies include: surveillance of blindness, development and implementation of national programmes, and development of primary eye care and trachoma control in the framework of primary health care.

The following are some examples of specific countries in which WHO and non-governmental organizations have been active during the past few years.

Afghanistan WHO staff and short-term consultants have assisted in planning and conducting surveys to assess the amount, distribution, and causes of blindness. A National Plan for the Prevention of Blindness has been prepared and submitted to the government for implementation. WHO-supported training courses for eye care personnel were held in Afghanistan as well as several other Middle-Eastern countries. Also, WHO fellowships were awarded to ophthalmologists from Afghanistan and other countries for training in public health ophthalmology.

Egypt WHO and the International Eye Foundation (IEF) have sponsored surveys to determine the causes of blindness in Egypt. These surveys have shown that cataract as well as trachoma are the major contributors to visual loss. The IEF also has completed a two-year project in Cairo, training health workers in primary eye care and blindness prevention. Over one million dollars worth of supplies and equipment were provided to the Ministry of Health for use in its ophthalmic programmes. In addition, IEF held the Fifth World Congress of the Society of Eye Surgeons in Cairo in 1984.

Jordan Jordan is among the countries collaborating with WHO in the development of plans to better integrate primary eye care and primary health care. The recently formed Jordanian National Committee for the Prevention of Blindness is playing a role in this activity. With support from WHO, a national seminar on blindness prevention was held in Amman in June of 1986.

Libya WHO collaborated in the development of a national plan for the prevention and control of impaired vision and blindness, with an emphasis on primary eye care and a comprehensive community-oriented programme integrated with primary health care. Also, WHO, is assisting in the planning of a survey to assess the causes and distribution of blindness in Libya.

Morocco   In Morocco, Helen Keller International (HKI) is collaborating with the ministry of health in the development of an intensive training programme to upgrade health workers' skills so that they can deliver eye care services to the Agadir region.

Oman   The national programme for trachoma control and the prevention of blindness, developed in collaboration with WHO, has been integrated into the new national health plan.

Pakistan   WHO is working with the newly formed national committee for the prevention of blindness to formulate a national programme. Of special concern is trachoma control and its integration with primary health care. Also, WHO is co-operating in a project for manpower training; courses have been held in Pakistan and several other countries. In addition, an ophthalmologist from Pakistan was among those granted WHO fellowships for training in public health ophthalmology. Also in Pakistan, the Royal Commonwealth Society for the Blind (RCSB) supports eye camps, and has contributed 50 per cent support for Layton Rahmatulla Benevolent Trust eye care programmes.

Saudi Arabia   With the support of the IEF and in consultation with WHO, Saudi Arabia has completed a major survey of the causes and distribution of eye disease. Cataract was found to be the leading cause of blindness, although trachoma is still a problem, particularly among people over age 60. The King Khaled Eye Specialist Hospital is the focal point for this nation-wide survey effort. In 1985, this hospital was designated as a WHO Collaborating Centre for the Prevention of Blindness.

Somalia   WHO, in collaboration with several non-governmental organizations, is assisting Somalia in the preparation of a national prevention of blindness programme.

Tunisia   In consultation with WHO, the national programme for the prevention of blindness has been elaborated to include plans for the integration of primary eye care and primary health care. Also, WHO-supported training courses have been held for health care workers essential to prevention of blindness programmes. With WHO support, a regional meeting on primary eye care was held in Tunis in December, 1985. Representatives of nine countries participated.

NORTH AMERICA

Helen Keller International

Bangladesh In 1984 the first evaluation of the country-wide vitamin A distribution programme in Bangladesh was completed. The study examined the nutritional status of 20 000 preschool children. Results showed that eight million, ages one through six, were receiving vitamin A capsules—a coverage rate of 46 per cent based on a target population of 20 million—and that no child who had received a capsule had gone blind. HKI's work in Bangladesh has been in collaboration with WHO, UNICEF, and other international agencies with funding from AID.

Fiji Since 1981 HKI has provided technical and material assistance to develop and implement primary eye health care. Nurses, health sisters, and tertiary level medical staff are trained in delivering basic and curative eye care. This work has relied on co-operation of AID, the Peace Corps, Christoffel-Blindenmission, the Royal Commonwealth Society for the Blind, Foresight, the Fiji Society for the Blind and Ministries of Education, Health, and Social Welfare.

Indonesia In the late 1970s, HKI with collaboration from WHO and UNICEF and funding from AID initiated the first major study of vitamin A deficiency. As a result, the Indonesian government established prevention of nutritional blindness as a major health priority. In 1981, in collaboration with the Indonesian government and the International Centre for Epidemiologic and Preventive Ophthalmology at Johns Hopkins University, HKI undertook a three-year survey in Aceh. The results suggested that even mild vitamin A deficiency is linked to child mortality.

Therefore, HKI continues to control blindness from vitamin A deficiency through the following activities: development of a risk index of vitamin A deficiency, integration of vitamin A into immunization programmes, activities in West Sumatra to increase coverage of supplemental vitamin A and increase the consumption of foods rich in vitamin A, fortification of monosodium glutamate (MSG) with vitamin A, and efforts to introduce liquid vitamin A supplementation as a routine part of the national family nutrition improvement programme. Training materials for health care workers, the organization of training courses, and the establishment of a system of low-cost eyeglass production are part of the primary eye care programme.

Morocco HKI has assisted in establishing an effective eye care delivery system through training health workers and hospital based nurses at the major hospital centre and includes identification and treatment of eye disease as well as referral of eye patients. Expansion from the hospital to rural satellite centres is planned.

Papua New Guinea In 1984, HKI began a pilot project to demonstrate the feasibility of community-based education/rehabilitation and primary eye care in selected target area.

Peru In 1982, with support of the Government's eye health programme through COLEB, a prevalence study to determine the major causes of blindness was undertaken. As a result, a plan to reduce the incidence of blindness through training primary health workers and general physicians in prevention, early detection, treatment, and referral of eye patients was undertaken. The programme includes manuals for use by health workers and public education messages shown in theatres, on television, and on radio.

Philippines Out of a population of 53 million, an estimated 800 000 persons are blind, giving the Philippines one of the highest rates of blindness in the world. In collaboration with the Philippines Eye Research Council, HKI has provided technical assistance in developing a programme to prevent blindness in two provinces in the Bicol region.

Sahel Region of Africa HKI has assembled three teams to perform assessments of nutritional blindness and trachoma among young children in the region to determine identification of target populations, extent of vitamin A deficiency and trachoma; identification of key intermediaries and a network for the distribution of vitamin A and tetracycline eye ointment; level of information available about vitamin A deficiency and trachoma and the need for training health workers. Following an evaluation of the results, HKI plans to implement programmes in the Sahel region.

Sri Lanka A primary eye care project was introduced in 1983 to provide training to public health nurses, inspectors, and family health workers, in the early detection, treatment, and referral of persons with eye problems. A programme of vision screening conducted by public health workers has been introduced into the school system. Eyeglasses are provided free of charge.

Sudan and Ethiopia High rates of xerophthalmia were discovered in the feeding centres in Ethiopia and in the children of Ethiopian refugees in Sudan. HKI developed training materials appropriate for health workers in order to implement a programme to provide vitamin A for the treatment and prevention of nutritional blindness in emergency situations. A total of 2 million vitamin A capsules have been distributed to feeding centres in Ethiopia for the prophylactic dosing of all children. Another half million doses of liquid vitamin A have been sent to refugee camps in Sudan through the United Nations High Commission for Refugees.

Tanzania In 1984, as part of an overall effort of the Ministry of Health in collaboration with the National Prevention of Blindness Committee, Christoffel-Blindenmission, and the Royal Commonwealth Society for the Blind, HKI began a programme in the Kongwa area of the Dodoma region of Northern Tanzania. The programme has concentrated on addressing the incidence of cataract, trachoma, and xerophthalmia, with particular emphasis on integrating a cost-effective primary eye care programme into the existing health care structure. The programme has established a system of cataract surgery that can be replicated in areas of scarce resources and has demonstrated the feasibility of a delivery system for the control of trachoma and infectious diseases. In collaboration with Johns Hopkins University and with funding from the Edna McConnell Clark Foundation, HKI completed in 1987 a major study of trachoma risk factors in central Tanzania. A further investigation will attempt to discover how the identified risk factors (flies near the doorway and dirty hands and faces) are related to the transmission of trachoma.

International Eye Foundation

Since 1983, the International Eye Foundation has been involved in a collaborative effort to establish a course of study for general practitioners from the Carribean leading to a Diploma in Ophthalmology at the Barbados campus of the University of West Indies. The objective of the programme is to train physicians from Dominica, Grenada, St. Lucia, St. Vincent, Belize, and Barbados so that they may provide qualified, regular eye care to their home islands.

The IEF has provided ophthalmic training to nurses working in relatively isolated island communities in hospital settings and among district nurses, family nurse practitioners, and community health workers located in rural areas. The Royal Commonwealth

Society for the Blind, Operation Eyesight Universal, and HKI collaborate with IEF in Carribean eye care projects.

The IEF continues its programme of service and training on the islands of Grenada and St. Lucia, the latter in collaboration with Massachusetts Eye and Ear Infirmary. Approximately 20 000 patients a year are seen and over 400 major surgeries performed on these two islands alone. In 1985, the IEF assumed responsibility for providing eye care on the islands of St. Kitts and Nevis. A glaucoma survey on the island of St. Lucia has been undertaken.

Dominican Republic   A two-year primary eye care programme was completed in 1985. This project involved training health personnel and educators, provided ophthalmic equipment to hospitals and ophthalmic aides to regional health centres and organizing teaching conferences for the ophthalmological society. The basics of eye care were taught to 500 physicians, 380 nurses, and 5900 health workers.

Puerto Rico   Since 1969, the IEF has provided fellowships to 500 Latin-American physicians to attend the University of Puerto Rico's basic ophthalmic science course.

Egypt   In 1984, the medical arm of IEF sponsored its Fifth World Congress in Cairo. Over 1000 ophthalmologists from around the world participated. The theme was ophthalmology and prevention of blindness in the developing world. In 1985, over 600 health workers received training in Cairo in primary eye care and blindness prevention. Surveys were conducted to determine the prevalence and etiology of blindness in rural and urban areas.

Guinea   A national ophthalmic referral centre in Conakry was refurbished and equipped by IEF.

Kenya   From 1977 to 1983, several hundred health workers have received training in primary eye care and prevention of blindness.

Honduras   In 1983, 1250 health care workers were trained in eye care and prevention of blindness. A laser has been provided to San Felipe Hospital and ophthalmologists trained to use it. Community health promoters in rural areas will be trained in eye care to handle the growing patient load.

Ecuador   Rural physicians and nurses will be trained in primary eye care and screening programmes developed.

Saudi Arabia IEF conducted a major study of blindness and eye disease in which 17 000 individuals were examined. This was done in conjunction with the King Khaled Eye Specialist Hospital and Ministry of Health.

Malawi In 1983, the first class of ophthalmic medical assistants graduated from the Southern African Sub-regional Ophthalmic Training Centre which emerged as a result of successful interagency co-operation including IEF, the Royal Commonwealth Society for the Blind, WHO, Operation Eyesight Universal, and the Government of Malawi. In 1983, during a three-month survey, over 7000 people were given complete ocular examinations and 50 000 children were examined for nutritional deficiencies.

Ethiopia The IEF in collaboration with Helen Keller International, the Ministry of Health and the faculty of medicine at Addis Ababa University will establish a one-year training programme to provide the Ministry of Health with primary eye care workers to work in unserved rural areas.

Zimbabwe In 1986, the IEF began a three-year project to assist the Ministry of Health in the development of an appropriate eye health care system. Ophthalmic medical assistants and general health workers will be trained in the provision of primary eye care at the rural and village levels.

Rotary International

Bangladesh Rotarians in Bangladesh and Australia are launching a project to organize 700 eye camps over the next five years. Approximately 10 000 patients will be examined at each camp. Treatment and surgery for cataracts will be done and glasses prescribed.

Dominican Republic A grant of US$227 000 is equipping an eye unit for the Diabetes Hospital in Santo Domingo. Nearly 70 000 patients are treated annually. Ongoing public education in the prevention of blindness from diabetes will be continued.

India Rotary funding began in 1980 with matching funds from the Canadian International Development Agency to immunize children in Southern India against measles. Also funded was a three-year medical training and development project in Amritsar, Punjab to provide sight restoration services to millions of cataract patients.

Mexico A grant of US$159 500 supports activities of Rotary clubs in Northern Mexico to provide eye examinations, eyeglasses, and medical eye care for low-income children and adults, also equipment, supplies, and a van for rural use. In addition to the above projects, Rotary funds child nutrition work in Guatemala, Honduras, Thailand, and Uganda.

Eye Care, Inc.

Eye Care, Inc., founded Eye Care Haiti (ECH), the largest provider of eye health services in Haiti which are supported generously by Christoffel-Blindenmission. A nation-wide network of ophthalmic assistants has been trained and certified to screen children and adults in remote areas. Signs of xerophthalmia, glaucoma, and eye infections are found and referred for medical care. ECH operates eight centres staffed by ophthalmologists and ophthalmic assistants for assessing visual acuity and evaluating and treating eye conditions. In addition, four major regional centres, three physician-staffed ophthalmology clinics and four satellite posts provide eye care to the most remote areas of Haiti. Community outreach involving primary health care services has served over 50 000 people in one location. ECH assisted with training physicians and other staff in eye care. The services of a teaching fellow in ophthalmology are provided to instruct residents at University Hospital and Jacomel Clinic. A project is underway to determine what proportion of personnel and resources to commit to each task performed by health workers and whether these resources might be more profitably spent if focused on high-risk mothers and children.

Seva Foundation

India Seva's support of Aravind Eye Hospital has subsidized 52 000 free cataract operations during the past five years; financed construction of a ward for non-paying patients; funded a free ward at a satellite eye hospital; provided consultants in hospital administration, health education, and epidemiology; provided a computer system to manage data; funded training in hospital administration; donated ophthalmic surgical supplies and equipment; aided in the development of research grants to increase the number of persons served; and established a microbiology lab.

Nepal Seva's nation-wide programme provides volunteer eye surgeons, administrative support, surgical supplies and equipment, training ophthalmic assistants, and support for start-up of indigenous eyeglass manufacturing. Since January 1984, Seva has sponsored all eye care services in Nepal's Lumbini Zone. Of Lumbini's 1.7 million people, roughly 40 000 are blind in one or both eyes. Approximately 133 000 (7.5 per cent) have potentially blinding trachoma. At least 700 children suffer from eye problems due to insufficient vitamin A. Eighty per cent of this blindness is preventable or curable through methods available in Nepal. The programme provides training and education to primary eye care volunteers and teachers. These are hospital-based services, eye camps, school screening programmes, and district clinics.

Canadian National Institute for the Blind

CNIB will urge the reactivation of a forum, such as a Canadian Co-ordinating Committee on Blindness Prevention and Sight Enhancement, to benefit concerned government and community organizations. The committee would be formed from a nucleus of national groups and organizations with opportunity for individual input. It would act as a single, powerful voice expressing the concerns of people who are threatened by blindness. It would promote initiatives in blindness prevention and sight enhancement.

The Secretariat of CNIB's E. A. Baker Foundation for Prevention of Blindness will provide consultation and funding for the production of educational material on blindness prevention assisted through the guidance of CNIB's National Communications Department. Research and training opportunities for those in the vision care field will be continued. Eye Bank programmes will remain within health-science facilities, with CNIB acting in a support role to provide education and promotion. Mobile eye equipment continues to extend services to Canadians in remote areas and the Federal/Provincial health safety net continues to ensure that Canadians can receive adequate eye care. Preschool, geriatric, and other vision screening programmes will remain the responsibility of the public health sector. CNIB will continue to encourage and promote, at the provincial level, the Wise Owl Club of Canada programmes that recognizes employers and employees whose safe practices have prevented serious eye injuries.

National Society to Prevent Blindness

The National Society to Prevent Blindness does not offer services or funding for programmes outside the continental United States. A brief summary of the recent activities in the United States follows.

In 1985, the National Society to Prevent Blindness embarked on nation-wide strategic planning—a process that studies the past, analyses the present in order to help the organization develop goals for the future. This plan has provided a focus for the Society for the next three years and defined its mission to preserve sight and prevent blindness. The Society's major programmes include:

1. Improving and maintaining the visual quality of life for older adults through education of the non-eye professions and the public about eye health needs of the ageing population.
2. Two Home Eye Tests—one for preschool children and the other for adults. The preschool test checks visual acuity while the adult test provides a check for signs of macular degeneration, glaucoma, and for near or far-sighted refractive errors.
3. A television eye test that permits viewers to test visual acuity and peripheral vision on their home TV screens. Merck, Sharp & Dohme International is making this test available in various languages.
4. Eye safety in sports through educating the professions and public about eye protection needed for sports such as tennis, squash, hockey, and handball.
5. Eye safety in industry through use of the Wise Owl Club. Membership is composed of men and women whose sight has been saved through eye protection during an accident.
6. Eye safety in the home and on the farm. Protection of vision against exploding batteries.
7. Establishment of self-help groups for glaucoma patients.
8. Data collection on causes of blindness.
9. Support of basic and clinical research grants with budgets limited to US$10 000 in the United States.

SOUTH ASIA

With the assistance of the World Health Organization (WHO) and a wide range of governmental and non-governmental organizations, the nations in this region are moving forward in assessing the prevalence and distribution of blinding diseases. Also, there has been great progress in the development of national plans and programmes, in the improvement of infrastructures for eye care, and in the integration of eye care services with primary health care.

Training programmes are increasing the number and quality of eye care personnel, including physicians, ophthalmic assistants, nurses, and community health workers. Research and technology development are also being fostered in this region. Activities in specific countries include the following.

Bangladesh Since 1978, Helen Keller International (HKI) has provided technical assistance to the vitamin A blindness prevention programme of the Government of Bangladesh. In 1984, HKI completed a major national nutritional blindness study, the first evaluation of the country-wide vitamin A distribution programme in Bangladesh. The study estimated that 46 per cent of the children in the target population were receiving vitamin A capsules, and yielded valuable data on the risk of vitamin A deficiency in various groups of children. With the collaboration of WHO and with financing from the US Agency for International Development, HKI is now engaged in a major blindness prevention and child survival campaign in Bangladesh.

Also, the Royal Commonwealth Society for the Blind (RCSB) and Operation Eyesight Universal (OEU) are supporting eye camps and other programmes in Bangladesh. These eye camps carried out more than 50 000 cataract operations last year. Also, Foresight of Australia, in co-operation with RCSB and Andheri Hilfe of West Germany, is supporting a major eye infirmary and training complex at Chittagong. Andheri Hilfe is also co-operating with the Bangladesh National Society for the Blind in a programme to treat curable blindness through newly established eye hospitals and travelling eye camps.

India With the support of WHO, the Aravind Eye Hospital and the Indian Government began a sight-restoration programme in the Maldive Islands. Under the Indo-US Science and Technology Initiative the National Eye Institute of the United States (NEI) is engaged in collaborative studies with three research institutions in India: nutritional blindness is being studied at the National Institute of Nutrition in Hydrabad, risk factors in age-related cataract is the subject of an NEI-supported case control study at the Dr Rajendra Prasad Centre for Ophthalmic Sciences in New Delhi, and Eales' disease is being investigated at the Madurai Kamaraj University and the Aravind Eye Hospital in Madurai. In addition, the NEI has contracted with the University of Michigan to provide consultation for a study of the barriers to cataract surgery.

RCSB has made a major investment in India, providing support for eye camps which in 1985 performed more than 211 000 cataract operations. Hospital construction, provision of mobile eye units, and projects on the prevention of xerophthalmia have also been among RCSB contributions. In addition, RCSB may fund a new International Centre for Community Ophthalmology in Tamil Nadu. RCSB also provided emergency assistance in Bhopal following the chemical disaster.

OEU has 30 programmes operating in India. These include eye hospitals, eye departments in general hospitals, ophthalmic clinics, eye camps, training programmes, nutritional programmes for the prevention of xerophthalmia, and a grassroots programme for the provision of ophthalmic care to all age groups of the population. Also, OEU is collaborating with RCSB to provide assistance to over 50 eye camps.

Seva Foundation has continued to support Aravind Eye Hospital, which has now grown into one of the premier eye care centres in the world. In 1985, more than 23 000 eye operations were performed at Aravind, and more than 230 000 patients were treated.

Foresight has established a clinic in Bombay to help people with low vision. Impact India, a national programme launched as part of the International Initiative Against Avoidable Disablement, is addressing nutritional blindness and cataract along with other disabling conditions.

Nepal A nation-wide survey conducted under the auspices of WHO indicated a great need for prevention of blindness initiatives in Nepal. In collaboration with WHO, Seva Foundation and Aravind Eye Hospital have assisted in the development of the Nepal Blindness Programme. The programme has strengthened eye care facilities, including rural eye care centres, and has trained ophthalmologists and ophthalmic assistants to staff them. Prevention of nutritional blindness is another component of the programme.

Sri Lanka HKI, in association with the Sarvodaya Shramandana Movement, is conducting a primary eye care programme in the Kurunegala District. The programme focuses on the training of health personnel in the early detection and treatment of people with eye problems. Also included is vision screening in schools in the project area. A rehabilitation project provides basic skills to blind people in rural communities.

SOUTH-EAST ASIA

With the support of the World Health Organization (WHO), large-scale surveys for the assessment of blindness at the national level have been conducted in several countries, including Indonesia, Burma, and Thailand. Initiatives to develop national plans in more countries of the region continue, but evaluative mechanisms have yet to be developed. An effort to strengthen eye health infrastructure is ongoing in Burma and Thailand, and referral systems have been developed in support of primary eye care services. In Burma, Indonesia, and Thailand more personnel are being trained in eye care. These training programmes are contributing to the enhanced implementation of programme activities at a national level. All countries in the region have already established training schemes. Research is being supported also; for example, a study of risk factors for blindness from angle-closure glaucoma is now being carried out in Rangoon, Burma.

Funds for the support of prevention of blindness activities in the region are being supported by a wide range of governmental and non-governmental organizations, including the United Nations agencies, AGFUND, the Japan Shipbuilding Industry Foundation, the Royal Commonwealth Society for the Blind (RCSB), the Christoffel-Blindenmission (CBM), the Asian Foundation for the Prevention of Blindness, and several others. Activities in specific countries include the following:

Burma A study of the prevalence and distribution of trachoma has provided the information needed to begin a major control effort.

Indonesia As a result of studies encouraged by WHO and supported by Helen Keller International (HKI) and the US Agency for International Development, Indonesia has established prevention of nutritional blindness as a major priority. HKI has assisted in design of a national control strategy and has worked with the Government of Indonesia to design and establish a surveillance system and to expand vitamin A capsule distribution, food fortification, and nutrition education. Recently, these programmes have received even greater emphasis because a three-year survey sponsored by HKI produced evidence that even mild vitamin A deficiency is linked to increased child mortality.

HKI's Indonesian project also involves promoting and developing primary eye care activities for the Indonesian Ministry of Health. Included are the development of local training materials for health care workers, the organization of training courses, and an effort to establish a system of low cost eyeglass production. The Society Against Blindness Overseas, of The Netherlands, is also contributing to blindness prevention programmes in Indonesia.

Malaysia   A WHO-sponsored seminar on the prevention of blindness took place in December 1986 in Kuala Lumpur. WHO is investigating a plan for eye care in a pilot programme of primary health care in the state of Sarawak. Also, RCSB is supporting a mobile eye unit and prevention of blindness activities in Malaysia.

Thailand   HKI is carrying out a project to improve educational and vocational opportunities for the blind in Thailand. The Government of Thailand, private sector organizations in that country, international technical assistance agencies, and several US corporations are contributing to this effort.

With the support of the US National Eye Institute, WHO has carried out a major study on utilization of eye health care in northern Thailand. This study, which is unique for a developing country, has proved valuable in demonstrating the social and economic aspects of the utilization of eye care services at various levels.

WESTERN PACIFIC

The Western Pacific region accommodates about one-third of the world's population and includes the most populous country in the world, China, as well as one of the smallest ones, Naul. Geographically, it includes such crowded countries as Japan and such diversified populations as the Western Pacific islands. Economically, this region includes both developed and developing countries, but in general it is better off than Africa or South-East Asia. The health status of the region, including vision problems and blindness, varies widely.

One of the first prevention of blindness activities at the regional level was the WHO-sponsored meeting in Manila in 1979. On that occasion an overall review was made of the ongoing activities in two WHO regions: South-East Asia and the Western Pacific. After discussing the future of national activities, plans were made for the WHO Regional Workshop of 1981. At this Manila meeting the member states discussed and agreed upon establishing national programmes in which primary eye care would be the core strategy.

Blindness prevention has a long history in this region. Trachoma control has existed in China, Vietnam, Japan, and many oth Western Pacific countries for a long time. In addition, the region', nutrition programmes have often included remedies to vitamin A deficiency. Health care in general seems to have recently come to a new stage where more emphasis is put on comprehensiveness and community participation. Primary health care is becoming a well-accepted concept.

This new trend in health care, which includes eye care, has generated a new start in this region, and in many countries prevention of blindness has now become an important part of the national health programme. This is well reflected in national programmes that have established a programme of basic eye care to all (the Primary Eye Care Approach), the elimination of endemic blindness, and the restoration of sight and/or rehabilitation.

Present situation of the blindness problem

Concrete epidemiological data on the magnitude of the problem of blindness in the region is still lacking. However, most countries have a blindness rate of approximately 0.5 per cent or even less. Nevertheless, there are still pockets where the rate is 1 per cent or more because of the lower level of socio-economic development, way of life, climate, and health care system of the countries. Highly industrialized countries in the region, such as Australia, New Zealand, and Japan have rates of about 0.2 per cent. However, they are facing a blindness problem of a different nature. China is said to have a blindness rate of perhaps 0.3 to 0.5 per cent.

Some distinctive trends regarding blindness in this region should be discussed. The major causes of blindness are shifting from those that are avoidable to those that are unavoidable, thus increasing the complexity of the problem and the difficulty of its control. For example, eye injuries in industry are more complicated and cause more corneal trauma and infection than those that happen during the performance of agricultural work. Proper eye care to address these problems will have to cover occupational and environmental health and be strongly linked with rehabilitation programmes.

The remarkable progress that has been seen in the health of the general population of the region is exemplified in a rapid fall in the infantile mortality rate and increased longevity. However, this has caused the elderly population to increase rapidly. Therefore, prevention of blindness related to ageing, especially to the problem of cataract, is becoming more important in all countries in this region.

However, the tragedies of social and political instabilities, refugee problems, and war are creating in some areas the need for eye care in the form of disaster management. Therefore, international aid must be continued for some time.

Major causes of blindness

Causes of blindness in the region of the Western Pacific appear nearly similar to those in the neighbouring region of South-East Asia. They are as follows:

Cataract

In many countries, cataract is by far the leading cause of blindness if untreated. As the ageing population increases, cataract in going to be the major target for prevention of blindness programme—a situation similar to other regions.

Xerophthalmia and keratomalacia

These conditions are still endemic in Laos, and they remain a potential threat in some countries such as the Philippines, Vietnam, and some South Pacific islands—especially in association with possible outbreaks of measles.

Trauma

This is the most important preventable cause of blindness among school-age children in all countries. In agricultural areas even minor injuries of the cornea may lead to blindness by infection after corneal trauma. Prevention of minor corneal injury is therefore important to prevention of blindness.

Special attention must be given to the rapid industrialization occuring in this region during recent years because such development often leads to increased work-place accidents that cause blindness. However, Japan's experience in the 1960s is encouraging. The number of occupational injuries, including those to the eye, has reduced markedly in Japan over the last three decades. This is the result of a combined approach that has included intensive education, law enforcement, first-aid training, provision of protective devices, and effective surveillance of work sites.

Trachoma

This condition, which was once the leading cause of blindness in China, has been brought under control by vigorous national efforts over the past several decades. In Vietnam, the trachoma control activities of the past 20 years are currently under assessment. Strong action seems necessary for Laos. Among the South Pacific islands its active form remains endemic in many areas; however, fewer complications are often manifested in cases there.

Ophthalmia neonatorum

Gonorrhoea and inclusion conjunctivitis in the newborn is said to be increasing in many countries, including Japan. Crédé's method of using antibiotics is widely used for the prevention of this condition, but a reassessment of the practices of birth attendants may also be needed.

Pterygium

It is indeed a tragedy that in some remote areas such easily cured blindness as that caused by pterygium is left untreated simply because of inadequate eye care. The condition is endemic in the South Pacific, the Philippines, and the Indo-China subregion. Provision of proper eye care, especially in outlying areas, is needed.

Glaucoma

Glaucoma poses a great challenge to prevention of blindness programmes. Because of scattered reports about the prevalence of different types of glaucoma, prevention programmes need to develop a sophisticated response to this disease. In glaucoma one eye often becomes blind while the other eye still provides useful vision, thus giving clinicians a chance of preventing total blindness from this disease. In the South Pacific glaucoma of any type is said to be rare among the indigenous population, whose intraocular pressure is usually low.

Malnutrition remains the cause of general health and vision problems in some famine areas of this region. In contrast, over-eating and excessive consumption of alcohol often pose health hazards in some South Pacific islands and affluent countries. Because a high prevalence of diabetes exists in the South Pacific, diabetic retinopathy plays a significant role in these islands, particularly Tahiti and Naoru. It is also the principal cause of new adult blindness in developed countries such as Japan and Australia.

Genetic drift and the isolation of some populations cause genetic eye diseases that are a major cause of blindness in some islands of the South Pacific. Reducing the isolation of these populations is a solution that will take some time.

In addition to these serious threats to eye health, the importance of visual disabilities from refractive errors and presbyopia must also be taken into account. Most countries need programmes that provide spectacles at affordable price—an essential public need in the region.

Special features of blindness control programmes

Most national programmes for prevention of blindness reflect individual national situations. As mentioned earlier in this report, the Western Pacific region is composed of countries widely different in socio-economic, geographic, and political conditions. Consequently, programmes for the prevention of blindness must show remarkable diversion, although primary eye care will be a common feature in all of them.

Far East

China WHO continues to provide health professionals with opportunities to learn within China. At a national seminar in 1985 groups discussed topics such as the managerial aspects of mass cataract intervention and low vision aids. Supplies and equipment are being supplied to primary eye care pilot programmes in such places as Huai-Lou County, near Beijing, and elsewhere.

Surveys on the prevalence and causes of blindness have been accomplished in a number of provinces. In many cases these have been followed by implementation of locally planned programmes for the prevention of blindness. The Epidemiological Study of Eye Diseases in Shun-Yi County, near Beijing, is attempting to ascertain the prevalence rates of blindness and major eye diseases, including cataract, amblyopia, trachoma, and glaucoma. The sample size for this study is 10 851, or 2.12 per cent of the target population, which is made up mostly of farmers. A coverage rate of above 95 per cent of the basic survey area was achieved by stratified and random cluster sampling. The socio-economic status of the region is in the upper–middle level when compared with the rest of China but most parts of this county still lack medical care. Although most people never see an ophthalmologist, there is a county hospital and two village clinics that treat eye problems and there are 10 doctors in the county.

Some provinces have shown remarkable success in blindness control. Perhaps one reason for their success is their administration: they have separate task forces attached to the Health Authority and assigned exclusively to these activities. In these provinces blindness caused by trachoma is no longer a problem, but they are still faced with new challenges from glaucoma, uveitis, and cataract—the main cause of blindness in many parts of the country. The solution to the cataract problem requires an increase in those able to provide eye surgery, more managerial competence, and socio-economic arrangements. There are excellent centres of eye health care in Beijing, Shanghai, Guang Zhou, Hubei, and many other cities that form a central core for prevention of blindness activities in China.

Japan The first workshop on the prevention of blindness at the national level was held in November 1984 as a joint activity between the Japanese Ophthalmologists Association and World Health Organization. It was primarily attended by Japanese professionals interested in blindness prevention. The current situation of neighbouring countries was also reported. The meeting encouraged new trends in Japan towards community- and prevention-oriented eye care.

The Japanese Society for the Prevention of Blindness has recently been reorganized and is in the process of reinforcing its financial and administrative capacities. The Japan Shipbuilding Industry Foundation continues to support prevention of blindness activities throughout the world through donations to WHO.

Korea The national programme began in 1983 with a five-year plan for a combination of various action components: primary eye care by public health nurse practitioners, especially in remote areas; the teaching of eye health in school; and instruction in eye care during maternity, in childhood, and within occupational health settings. WHO has supported annual workshops and research into improving refraction services for school children, including the feasibility of supplying low-cost spectacles. Blindness in Korea seems no longer a major health issue, perhaps because the promotion of eye health has been stressed in their national programme. In fact, the Korean programme is considered a model to other rapidly progressing countries in the region.

Indo-China

Vietnam WHO has helped Vietnam's national programme of trachoma control to become more comprehensive and to include a wider range of problems. In addition to supplying equipment, technical assistance was provided in 1985 to help organize a national seminar on eye health planning in Ho Chi Minh City. Later that year specialists were sent by WHO to help prepare the first five-year plan of primary eye care programmes for selected provinces.

Noting that trachoma control in Vietnam has achieved good results, WHO has provided funds for several programme evaluations and for the development of a permanent evaluation mechanism for Vietnam's entire blindness prevention programme. Although this national programme has been very promising; additional support would encourage further progress.

Laos   Although blindness prevention is a high priority in this country, malnutrition remains endemic, infectious diseases are not entirely under control, and eye care is almost non-existent—there is one tertiary centre.

Collaboration with WHO resulted in a national seminar in October 1986 that drew up a five-year plan for establishing an eye care network covering a population of 3 million in the five provinces along the Mekong River. Each year in one of the designated provinces one tertiary and two secondary eye care centres are to be built. In addition, there will be primary eye care training at the secondary centres.

Democratic Kampuchea   Currently no information is available regarding the situation of eye care in this country.

Oceania

Fiji   Fiji was the first of the South Pacific islands to institute a national eye care programme in 1983. The current level of eye care in Fiji has resulted from the training of mid-level health workers in primary eye care. In parallel, ophthalmology training is underway at the eye unit of the teaching hospital in Suva so that specialized eye care can be provided at all divisional and selected subdivisional hospitals.

Trachoma, once regarded as the leading cause of blindness, declined and now the major problems seem to be cataract and glaucoma. However, trachoma still remains a health concern in some areas.

Oceania seems to require a sort of subregional programme in which Fiji could play a significant role in technical co-operation between countries.

Vanuatu   This country consists of seven islands located close together and inhabited by a population of 150 000, mostly

Melanesians. A primary eye care course and training by tutors was held in 1983. Specialized eye care is being provided by an Australian team that visits the area from time to time. A relatively well-developed health care infrastructure and enough expatriate physicians cover almost the whole country, but Fiji needs at least one full-time ophthalmologist.

Tonga Primary health care in this country of 90 000 inhabitants was started through WHO's assistance. The tertiary centre, which is served by one ophthalmologist needs to be strengthened by enlarging its capacity to provide care as well as training.

The geographical distribution of these islands does not seem to prevent easy referral from outlying islands to the centre. However, better primary eye care should be aimed at. Local capabilities should be improved to provide better basic eye care and an effective information system that can facilitate efficient specialized eye care, including referrals, and regular mobile services.

Samoa The situation of this nation of 300 000 is similar to Tonga regarding health care and the country's commitment to the health of its people. Primary eye care will be incorporated into the national programme, which will be expected to start soon. A strong tertiary centre already exists at the central hospital, which is served by two ophthalmologists.

Kiribati This nation consists of a number of small atolls scattered over a huge oceanic area where the international date line and the equator intersect. It has a population of 60 000, mostly Micronesians. This nation seems to require the inclusion of primary eye care to the ongoing primary health care programme. A major problem is its geography, which necessitates long distance referrals. The solution is to provide strong local capabilities for eye care on individual islands.

Trachoma has been found to be prevalent, and subclinical vitamin A deficiency is also a problem. An Australian team provides mobile services. However, the country wishes a gradual transfer of new technology, such as that used in cataract surgery, to local providers.

WHO is fully committed to assist the countries in this subregion to establish effective primary health care programs. Although progress seems substantial, further technical inputs in primary eye care are necessary to improve prevention of blindness activities in this subregion. Co-ordination of the activities of national governments, WHO, and non-governmental organizations is the essential

key to the successful development of prevention of blindness programmes in the Western Pacific region.

Australia   Australia is a sophisticated country with high technology and professional skills. The Australian Government is committed to assisting developing countries in the region giving high
priority to primary health care projects. The Government gives
more aid to nations in Oceania than any other nation.

Prevention of blindness funding

Initial funding for prevention of blindness activities in rural
Australia came principally through the Federal Government but
increasingly the programmes have been conducted through the individual states of Australia. Funding for overseas prevention of blindness comes from two sources:

1. Bilateral aid sources—the Australian Government has a heavy
   commitment to overseas aid in Oceania. The money being given
   by the Australian Government is in response to an approach at
   the government to government level. Some of this money is used
   in health care and prevention of blindness programmes.
2. Foresight   Australia—Australia's   only   international   non-
   governmental organization whose sole objective is overseas prevention of blindness. Foresight works in non-governmental
   organization partnership arrangement with the Royal Commonwealth Society for the Blind (RCSB), Helen Keller International,
   International Eye Foundation, and Operation Eyesight Universal. Foresight's annual budget has gradually increased and has
   tripled in the last eight years.

Prevention of blindness activities

The National Trachoma and Eye Health Programme identified the
important cause of blindness in rural Australia, particularly
amongst members of the 200 000 aboriginal population. The principal causes were cataract and external eye disease, in which
trachoma was a prominent factor.

Currently the Rural Eye Health Programmes have become the
responsibility of state committees which have a majority membership of aborigines and community groups with participation of
ophthalmologists on a state by state basis. Priorities are determined by each state committee, the programmes are costed and a

budget submitted. The mechanism is in keeping with the philosophy of the Federal Government and the eye profession that responsibility for eye care in the rural sector be determined by the recipients.

Urban prevention of blindness activities

The Australian Foundation for Prevention of Blindness in different states of Australia together with Lions Clubs are involved in programmes screening for glaucoma and visual defects in childhood. In Western Australia and New South Wales, screening programmes for the whole state have been undertaken to also survey diabetes and glaucoma. The screening programmes apart from identifying eye disease, are seen as an important means of increasing community awareness of eye health.

The Royal Australian College of Ophthalmologists has been active in drawing public attention to the importance of seat belts in motor vehicles to avoid eye injuries, as a result of road trauma. It has campaigned actively also to control the sale of fireworks and to encourage safety in sport and industry, emphasizing the importance of safety glasses.

Prevention of blindness overseas

Australia has an active programme of exchange of health personnel both for in-country training but also for work experience in Australia, particularly for individuals from the Asia-Pacific area, including Papua New Guinea, Fiji, Tonga, Singapore, Thailand, Bangladesh, and China. It recognizes the training and diplomas should be developed as far as possible in each country where the service is given in order to build national confidence and pride, and to increase the chances that those trained will ultimately practice in their own country.

Cataract surgical programmes have been conducted in Oceania through Aspect under the leadership of Dr J. Galbraith, particularly in the Solomon Islands, until more recently when the team included Tonga in their programme. Australia is also involved in prevention of blindness programmes in Papua New Guinea, Fiji, Solomon Islands, Tonga, Western Samoa, China, and Bangladesh, through the activities of Foresight.

6

Operations research in cataract blindness prevention

Leon B. Ellwein and *Carl Kupfer*

INTRODUCTION

Operations research can be defined as the application of analytical methods designed to help a decision-maker choose between various courses of action to accomplish specific objectives. Operations research uses the scientific method rather than using intuition, analogy, or trial and error in addressing problems involving people and material resources. Scientific methodology has traditionally been applied to the study of problems in the natural sciences. Operations research uses it in the study of man–machine systems. It is research applied to operational and management problems.

Its origins are linked to research on operational problems faced by the British military during World War II: they turned to scientists for aid in incorporating the then new radar into tactics for defence against the German air attack and in developing search strategies for detecting submarines that were threatening convoy shipping routes. For many operational problems, it is possible to develop a mathematical model of the system under study, and thus, through analytical simulation, one can test various solutions prior to their actual implementation. The classes of problems for which mathematical models have been successfully developed include those involving queuing, inventory, transportation, routing, and scheduling.[1] Queuing problems entail balancing the cost of service and the cost associated with waiting for service, for example determining an optimal balance between the number of examination stations in a busy clinic and the waiting time experienced by those being served. Inventory problems address trade-offs between the costs of storing goods and penalties associated with shortages. Transportation problems arise wherever one is faced with determining optimal shipping patterns, such as in allocating the production from several limited capacity facilities to satisfy the demand of geographically dispersed consumers while minimizing total transportation costs. Routing problems occur, for example, where one is concerned with finding the shortest route from an origin to a destination through a connecting network. Scheduling problems arise in settings where it is necessary to sequence a series of work tasks so that specified completion times can be met as, for example, in a medical service laboratory. Scheduling is complicated when there are a diversity of competing work orders with variability in processing times and the possibility of unanticipated interruptions.

Within the last two decades, operations-research concepts and techniques have been introduced to researchers and managers in health care delivery,[2] including those whose particular interests lie with primary health care problems faced by developing countries.[3]

In employing the scientific method, we pay particular attention to stating explicitly all assumptions and procedures used in data manipulation so that results are reproducible. Quantitation is always a hallmark characteristic. Because operational-research problems generally do not follow any one discipline, operations-research teams are frequently interdisciplinary, including where appropriate experts from such fields as medicine, statistics, behavioural science, physics, and engineering. Interdisciplinary teams provide the perspective that is necessary in addressing problems that are by nature multi-dimensional. The viewpoint of operations research is one of management, focused on decision-making and resource allocation. The viewpoint is prospective and not that of retrospective assessment and evaluation. It gives emphasis to addressing the whole problem with careful consideration of interactions between the component parts of the system being studied.

THE OPERATIONS-RESEARCH APPROACH

Although operations research follows generally accepted scientific methods familiar to those active in biomedical research, it is of value to discuss the methodology when it is adapted to new problem settings. Table 6.1 identifies three major phases of operations research.

Operations research begins with *problem analysis*, with the purpose of establishing a clear, unambiguous identification or characterization of the problem being faced. In biomedical research, problem analysis is a primary focus, where we stress studies of disease causation and the building of a knowledge base sufficient to provide leads for subsequent development of preventive or therapeutic interventions. Similarly, in patient management, we frequently spend a considerable amount of time and effort in diagnosis, which too is focused on problem identification. Problem identification can require a considerable amount of effort, including collection and analysis of background data. The underlying problem may not be readily apparent, and we must ensure that we are addressing the real problem rather than some false perception. It is difficult, if not impossible, to get the 'right' answer by addressing the 'wrong' problem.

Solution development is the second phase in operations-research endeavors. In the development of problem solutions, the first step is the definition of solution objectives, which may be expressed in terms of achieving certain extremes, such as minimizing the cost per case of blindness prevented or maximizing the number of cataract operations per year. Solution objectives reflect the desired consequences or impacts being sought, where the degree of achievement is subject to resource allocations or actions within the control of the decision-maker, such as the assignment of a particular treatment regimen to a disease diagnosis. In reference to biomedical research, such as that directed toward the development of a new drug, objectives are also clearly defined using measurable end-points focused on either the cure or reduction in morbidity of a defined disease problem.

In defining solutions objectives, we focus on measurability because we must be able to determine quantitatively the extent to which alternative solution approaches produce the desired outcome. Solution objectives serve as effectiveness measures only when properly stated. To ensure realism in defining solution objectives, we should make explicit those limitations on available resources or other natural limits that must be adhered to in optimizing achievement of objectives.

Table 6.1 Operations-research approach

Problem analysis
   Problem identification

Solution development
   Definition of solution objectives
   Formulation of alternatives
   Analysis of alternatives

Solution validation
   Testing of chosen alternative(s)
   Monitoring and evaluation

The second step in solution development entails the formulation of solution alternatives. This step is directed toward the question of 'What is the best way to achieve our objectives and, thereby, solve the problem being addressed?' This step is a creative, imaginative process. Theoretically, a very large number of solution possibilities exist, yet we are interested in only the one or a select few, that is most effective in achieving our objective. In generating alternative solutions, we can focus immediately on the formulation of a few good solution alternatives; or we can follow a process where we eliminate a large number of infeasible or poor alternatives while screening for the few worthy of further consideration. For example, in formulating patient education strategies we could begin by attempting to improve what currently is being done, or we could start at a general, and more generic level, by reviewing approaches used in non-medical settings until we find one or two that appear adaptable to our setting.

Whatever process we follow in the formulation of solution alternatives, we must make sure that the focus is on the identified problem and the associated solution objectives. We must make sure that any assumptions pertaining to the solution alternative are clearly stated and that the key features of any alternative are adequately described. As in the problem identification step, we may require investigative studies and gather pertinent data to provide leads that aid in solution formulation. For example, if we are dealing with medical treatment, we may wish to understand the mechanism-of-action of a existing chemotherapeutic agent so that we can design an improved drug. Fortunately, it has been possible to conduct such research and formulate effective preventive and therapeutic compounds without completely understanding the mechanisms involved, for example, with some common immunizations.

The third step in solution development entails the analysis of solution alternatives. Alternatives are analysed to estimate the extent to which they can be expected to achieve solution objectives, i.e. analysis of effectiveness. Each solution alternative is also analysed from the perspective of feasibility, for example to ensure that it does not violate resource constraints. Estimation of the cost that will be incurred in implementing each alternative is another important part of the analysis. Finally, we may wish to undertake sensitivity analysis, where we measure the sensitivity of the achievement of objectives to changes in assumptions, constraints, etc.

It should be noted that for many of the classic operations-research problems referred to in the Introduction, the three steps of solution development are completely integrated. In these cases we construct a model where the solution objective and resource constraints are stated as mathematical functions of the decision variables, and then sophisticated analytical methods are used to compute the best, or optimal, solution alternative.

The third phase in operations research is *solution validation*. This phase encompasses two steps. The first is field testing of the solution alternatives considered to be comparably effective. Testing of alternative solutions requires careful design to enable the decision-maker to ultimately choose between them. The study design may take the form of an experimental comparison, where the methods of randomized clinical trials are directly applicable. The scope of the field test should be limited, yet consistent with examining all questions and providing a reality test of critical assumptions. If the field test is directed toward validation of a single, preferred approach, a small-scale pilot test may suffice in confirming the soundness of previous analytical evaluations and assumptions. In either case, the details of testing methods and procedures must be clearly spelled out in a manual of operations and field personnel trained if the pilot test entails activities different from their usual job. Further, in instances where the alternative solution approach requires interface with some existing infrastructure, its integration as a part of the overall system must receive adequate consideration.

The second and final step in solution validation deals with monitoring and evaluation. As the field test is actually conducted, operations management is critical to assuring that the test protocol is carried out as designed—an important quality assurance function. Protocol adherence is necessary if we are to accurately assess the true potential of the alternative. This step includes data collection, analysis, and interpretation of field test results to measure effectiveness and the estimated costs of full-scale implementation. Conclusions based on the results of the field trial experience must be drawn and recommendations made to management. Documentation of testing results is particularly important where the solution alternative will be communicated to others for widespread application.

The phases and steps of the operations-research approach as detailed above are presented in a sequential, once through, fashion. It should be recognized that, in practice, these steps are more likely to be iterative, where the alternative formulation, analysis, testing, and evaluation cycle continues until the desired result is finally achieved.

BLINDNESS PREVENTION FROM A SYSTEMS PERSPECTIVE

As we address the blindness problem from a systems perspective, several facets become important in exploring problem identification and opportunities for solution development. Depending on specific circumstances, the problem and its potential for solution may lie within any one of the following: the biological process underlying the development of blindness, the behaviour of individuals affected, the existence of an intervention technology, or finally, the deployment of delivery system resources.

Let us consider these four facets in greater detail in the context of cataract blindness. As shown in Fig. 6.1, the biological problem

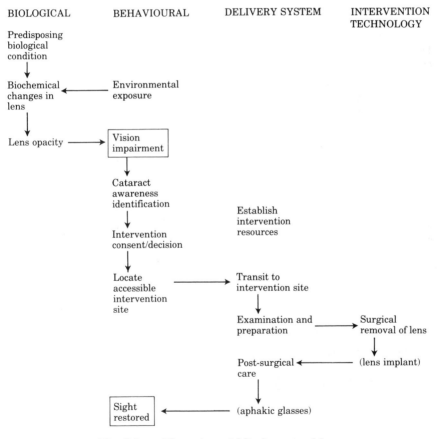

Fig. 6.1   The cataract blindness problem

manifests itself initially as a biochemical reaction perhaps leading to oxidative damage within the lens of the eye, possibly contributing to this change are genetic or other predisposing biological conditions within the host and exposure to causative agents or environmental conditions associated with host behaviour. These biochemical changes lead to lens opacity, a condition that results in vision impairment.

Vision impairment inevitably will impact upon the behaviour of the individual. Eventually the individual is expected to become aware of his vision impairment and whether it is affecting adversely the daily routine of living. Through health education, perhaps, it will be recognized that the decreased vision is due to cataract and that something can be done about it. After this identification, the individual must decide whether he is going to take action by seeking surgical intervention. The intervention decision is followed by the locating of an accessible intervention site. Without reasonably convenient access to intervention, even the most motivated individual may be deterred in seeking intervention.

The delivery system is accessed as the patient travels to a hospital-based intervention site or as the intervention delivery team comes to him, for example, in surgical eye camps where the intervention technology is brought to the patient's community. The delivery system includes a complete patient eye examination and, where indicated, preparation for cataract surgery. The pivotal intervention technology is the surgical procedure itself, the technology for the safe removal of the cataract lens. As noted in Fig. 6.1, this technology requires prerequisite resources in the form of trained ophthalmic surgeons, support personnel, surgical supplies, equipment, and facilities. These resources must be available within the delivery system if the curative intervention technology is to have a beneficial impact. After surgery, the delivery system is called upon for post-surgical care and aphakic correction.

Finally, the individual experiences restoration of sight, and the biological disease process has been overcome. The individual reaches this situation only after successfully passing through the prerequisite events. The individual must have: (a) identified his condition of vision impairment and recognized that something could be done about it, (b) made a decision to seek intervention, (c) been able to identify an accessible intervention site, and (d) expended the funds and other resources required to enter a delivery system that includes the surgical intervention technology of proven effectiveness.

In reviewing the cataract blindness problem from this perspective, we note first that current technology does not allow us to reverse, slow down, or prevent cataract formation. Solution development based on cataract prevention will be held in abeyance until further epidemiological and biochemical research, presently focused on problem identification and characterization, provides information on risk factors and disease etiology. Epidemiological surveys have revealed that cataract is relatively common and that in many countries a large number of people are experiencing advanced visual impairment despite the existence of an effective intervention. There is a disconcertingly large backlog of cataract blind individuals, even in countries where adequate numbers of trained manpower exist. (For example, India has 6000 ophthalmologists. If we assume that only 3000 of these operate on cataract cases and that each carries a realistic load of 100 cases per month for 10 months of the year, we would have 3 million cases operated per year throughout the country. This number is almost triple the amount of surgery currently being done.)

There are at least three factors contributing to this situation, all falling within the behavioural and delivery system portions of Fig. 6.1. First, we may need a redeployment of personnel and resources: the geographic distribution of ophthalmologists and other surgical resources generally does not follow the distribution of the population. Secondly, a number of cataract blind are not coming to surgery either because of a lack of awareness or because of no desire to seek surgery; these behavioural barriers include ignorance, fear of the unknown, ambivalence, and the attitude that fate is responsible for their condition and it would be unwise to change it. Thirdly, there are others who would seek surgery were it possible to reduce logistic and other economic-related barriers associated with the delivery system—beyond those associated with access to a maldistributed system. Cost barriers can, indeed, be significant and include not just out-of-pocket expenses for transportation, supplies, glasses and, possibly, the surgical procedure and post-surgical care, but also the lost earnings of a friend or family member accompanying the patient.

The specifics of behavioural and delivery system problems are likely to differ between cultures and countries, precluding the development of a single solution suitable for global application. Fortunately, this same degree of heterogeneity does not exist for problem analysis and solution development efforts dealing with the biological or anatomical system itself, such as is the case with biomedical research focused on development of prevention or treatment technologies. For example, the surgical technique for lens removal is equally applicable to all populations. Although behavioural and delivery system problems can require unique man-machine systems solutions, these problems can be addressed and solutions designed using common scientific methods as outlined above.

ARAVIND OPERATIONS-RESEARCH PROJECT

The Aravind Eye Hospital has been concerned with why rural people in Southern India facing cataract blindness do not come to surgery. Particularly those within reasonable distance of Madurai, where both Aravind and a government hospital provide cataract surgery without cost to the patient. Dr Venkataswamy, the Hospital Director, in collaboration with Dr Girija Brilliant, a health education specialist, conducted a preliminary study to investigate the barriers to cataract surgery.[4] As in a similar study in Nepal,[5] they learned that economic factors, such as cost of transportation, food during hospitalization, and lost earnings, as well as psychosocial factors such as lack of accompaniment, fear of surgery, and waiting for the lens to 'mature' were responsible for keeping visually impaired people away from cataract surgery. In collaboration with personnel from the University of Michigan, the University of Nebraska, and the National Eye Institute, National Institutes of Health an operations research study is being undertaken to investigate the effectiveness of alternative solutions to these barriers. Table 6.2 outlines this study using the framework of the operations-research approach.

Four alternative solution approaches were formulated, each with the objective of maximizing the percentage of cataract blind coming to surgery in rural areas of Southern India. The alternative solution approaches entail: (1) an aphakic motivator (an individual who has successfully undergone cataract surgery) going door-to-door within a village convincing those with visual impairment, thought to be due to cataract, to come to Aravind Hospital for examination and free surgery; (2) a health worker with six weeks of specialized ophthalmic training going door-to-door within a village to convince those determine to be cataract blend to come for examination and free surgery; (3) a screening van visiting a village with ophthalmic examination of all those coming for screening and referral to the hospital for surgery of all those who appear to be determined to have cataract blindness; and (4) the development of video messages that play in centrally located village markets encouraging those with blindness to seek examination.

Comparative effectiveness is being field tested in an experimental

Table 6.2 Aravind operations-research project

Problem: Behavioural and economic barriers to cataract surgery
Objective: Maximize percentage of cataract blind coming to surgery

Alternative solutions	*Alternative testing*
Aphakic motivator	Experimental comparisons—randomization of villages
–Door-to-door survey identification	Detailed operations manual
–Persuasion to obtain surgery decision	Personnel training
	Existing health system for surgery
Health worker	Pretesting of operations and data collection forms
–Door-to-door survey identification	
–Education to obtain surgery decision	*Monitoring and evaluation*
Screening van	Effectiveness evaluation
–Self-identification	–Experimental and control villages
–Publicity to obtain screening examination decision	–Based on surgical coverage
	–Door-to-door evaluation survey
Marketplace media	–Ophthalmologica examination
–Self-identification	
–Publicity to obtain examination decision	Cost analysis
	–Personnel
All alternatives	–Facilities
–Free travel, examination, surgery, post-operative stay, food, and glasses vs. only free examination, surgery, post-operative stay, and glasses	–Equipment
	–Materials
–Intra-capsular lens extraction	–Purchased services
	–Beneficiary costs

study design that includes randomized assignment of entire villages to each of the four intervention approaches. The study entails 100 villages with a total population of nearly 200 000 and an estimated cataract blindness prevalence of 2000 cases. Detailed operations manuals and training regimens have been prepared with extensive pretesting prior to implementation of the formal field trial. Pretesting led to improvements in training procedures, data collection forms, and the operations protocol. Existing health care delivery resources are being used for all surgical operations and post-surgery hospitalization at either the Aravind Eye Hospital, one of its satellite hospitals, or at the government hospital in Madurai.

The key evaluation index is surgical coverage, the percentage of those cataract blind that come to surgery because of the barrier reduction interventions. Evaluation entails a post-study visit to each village within the study population, where a survey team will go door-to-door to identify all aphakics and those with remaining visual impairment for examination by an ophthalmologist. In addition to those villages assigned to either of the barrier reduction approaches, control villages will also be examined. These control villages are needed so that the impact of the barrier interventions can be compared with doing nothing.

Another important part of the evaluation phase is the monitoring and analysis of the costs of conducting each of the four intervention approaches. Costs of personnel, facility equipment, supplies, and travel, whether incurred by the Aravind Hospital, donated by the villages, or incurred by the patient, will be recorded for each of the interventions during field testing. Cost-effectiveness of each of the four intervention approaches will be compared in the determination of the optimal solution approach.

Examining this project in terms of the cataract-blindness problem as outlined in Fig. 6.1, we find that, in cataract awareness/identification, the screening van and mass media rely on patient self-identification, whereas the aphakic motivator and health worker interventions entail identification by exhaustive household survey. With regard to consent/decision, the screening van and mass media interventions rely upon the influence of health-oriented publicity campaigns delivered on a community wide basis: aphakic motivator and health worker interventions involve person-to-person persuasion and health education. The delivery system includes a comparison between patient-arranged transportation and patient-supplied food versus free transportation and food. Half of the villages will be offered the free package. All patients will be offered free ophthalmic examination, surgery, and aphakic glasses.

Also, the anticipated five—seven-day post-operative hospital stay is provided without cost to the patient. Intra-capsular lens extraction will be used as the surgical technology for all patients.

As illustrated by the Aravind project, operations-research methods provide a scientific framework within which the cataract-blindness backlog can be addressed. Recognizing that the nature of the specific problem and corresponding solution approaches will differ from country to country, many such projects are called for. In some countries, the proper focus will be the behavioural features of the population; in others it will be the costs associated with the delivery system. Still in other countries, the first attack on the backlog problem will require solutions to the virtual absence of intervention resources, including trained ophthalmic personnel. Whatever the scenario, we advocate the methods of science in both problem identification and resolution as intuition, trial and error, and analogy are likely to produce many unproductive and false starts. The validity of barrier intervention methods and resource allocation schemes proposed as cost effective solution approaches must be scientifically established before widespread application is advocated. Anecdotal evidence produced under undefined conditions is to be viewed with scepticism.

Acknowledgments

This chapter is an expansion of that presented at the Third General Assembly of the International Agency for the Prevention of Blindness in New Delhi, 9 December 1986. Dr Ellwein was supported in part by National Eye Institute contract NO1–EY–5–2104. Acknowledgment is given to the clerical assistance of Cheryl Kibler.

References

1. Hillier, F. S. and Lieberman, G. J. (1986). *Introduction to operations research* (4th edn). Holden-Day, San Francisco.
2. Flagle, C. D. (1973). Operations research in the medical field. *Medical Progress Through Technology (Berlin)* 2, 7–12.
3. Blumenfeld, S. N. (1985). *Operations research methods: A general approach in primary health care.* PRICOR, Chevy Chase, Maryland.
4. Venkataswamy, G. and Brilliant, G. E. (1981). Social and economic barriers to cataract surgery in rural south India: A preliminary report. *Visual Impairment and Blindness*, pp.405–8.
5. Brilliant, G. E. and Brilliant, L. B. (1985). Using social epidemiology to understand who stays blind and who gets operated for cataract in a rural setting. *Social Science and Medicine (Oxford)*, 21, 553–8.

7

Mobilizing resources and political will: Convincing governments that prevention of blindness is cost-effective

Michael F. Drummond

INTRODUCTION

In most countries the resources for providing health care are increasingly stretched in the face of competing demands for their use. Technological advances in medicine have increased the range of treatment possibilities. At the same time changing public expectations have increased the demand for a greater range and quality of health services.

Against this background, those arguing for more funds to be devoted to eye health care increasingly need economic data in support of their claims. Although the specific issues vary from country to country the basic principles are the same, whether one is seeking to justify the fee schedule for cataract operations in a developed country, or seeking funds to perform more operations at US$25 per eye in a developing country where the annual per capita health care expenditure is only US$5.

THE ECONOMIC BURDEN OF ILLNESS

Investments in health care have typically been justified in economic terms by pointing to the economic burden of illness. The traditional approach to estimating the economic impact of ill health is to undertake a 'cost of illness' study of the type pioneered by Rice in the United States.[1] Here the cost of an illness, or group of illnesses, is considered to comprise the *direct* medical care costs, the *indirect* costs in terms of production losses owing to morbidity or premature mortality, and the *intangible* costs associated with morbid events. Typically, the intangible *costs are not estimated* owing to measurement difficulties and this may be a problem if these do not mirror the quantifiable costs.

Variations on this approach have been used to justify expenditure on eye care. For example, Bernth-Petersen[2] argued that in Denmark cataract surgery could be justified in terms of savings of other expenditure, estimating that the effect of the 3000 first eye cataract extractions performed in 1980 was to save around 400 places in nursing homes.

However, economists have become increasingly critical of traditional cost of illness studies. First, it could be considered to be a circular argument to suggest that priorities for future health care expenditures should follow the patterns currently observed in the cost of illness. Secondly, the analysis is biased against groups like the elderly or unemployed, as the indirect costs of illness for these individuals will be low. Thirdly, the intangible costs of illness may not mirror the direct and indirect costs. For example, two Gallop polls in the United States taken a decade apart, found that the two most feared diseases were cancer and blindness, although neither of these features in the top three places in most cost of illness rankings. Fourthly, cost of illness studies do not address whether effective interventions exist to combat the illnesses in question. A health problem may rank highly in terms of its economic impact, but no means may be available to tackle it. Conversely, a simple, quick and effective intervention may be available to tackle an illness further down in the ranking, such as cataract.

Finally, there are additional difficulties in applying the cost of illness methodology in the developing country context. First, because there may be no health care infrastructure to treat many illnesses, the direct costs, as traditionally measured, will be small. Rather, the economic impact of ill health will be on the families of the sufferers. Secondly, in a subsistence rural economy much production, and consequently production losses, may not be captured by examining the market wage rates of those in paid employment.

In fact the main *economic* benefits from investments in health care relate to the impact on the quality of life of the patient and his family, not to the factors typically measured in cost of illness studies. Ideally, we require a methodology that considers all the relevant benefits of health care interventions and compares them to the costs. Interventions could then be ranked in terms of their relative costs and benefits.

METHODS FOR ASSESSING THE COSTS AND BENE-FITS OF HEALTH CARE PROGRAMMES

The main justification for such analyses is, therefore, that the resources for the provision of health care are scarce, in that there are not, and never will be enough resources to satisfy human wants completely. All the methods of economic evaluation have the common feature that some combination of the inputs to a health care programme are compared with some combination of the outputs (see Fig. 7.1). The measurement of inputs, and their translation to money values, is relatively uncontroversial. However, the outputs can be assessed in a number of ways. First, they can be measured in the most convenient natural units (effects), such as 'years of life gained', 'number of fully immunized children', or 'cases successfully treated'. A study measuring outputs in this way would be called a cost-effectiveness analysis.

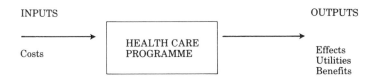

Fig. 7.1 Economic evaluation of health care programmes. (Source: Drummond *et al.* 1986.[5]

Secondly, the outputs can be measured in quality-adjusted life-years (QALYs), where the life extension gained is adjusted by a series of 'utility' weights reflecting the relative value of one health state compared to another. This approach is particularly useful where the success of a health care programme is more appropriately assessed in terms of *quality*, not quantity, of life gained. For example, Fig. 7.2 shows QALYs gained by cataract operation with and without resulting life extension. Anecdotal evidence suggests that in developing countries, individuals' lives might be extended by the operation if this increases mobility or enables the individual to support himself and his family better economically. A study measuring outputs in QALYs would be called a *cost-utility analysis*. (Some authors just view this as a special form of cost-effectiveness analysis.)

Finally, the outputs of health care programmes can be measured in money terms, so as to make them completely commensurate with the costs. Some categories of benefit are fairly easy to assess in this way but others, such as the value to the patient of feeling healthier,

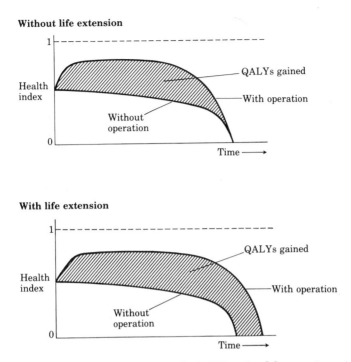

Fig. 7.2   Quality-adjusted life-years (QALYS) gained from cataract

are obviously more difficult to express in money terms, although such measurements are sometimes attempted. The practical limitations of this approach, known as *cost-benefit analysis*, have led to an increased popularity of cost-effectiveness and cost-utility analysis.

Economic evaluation has been widely applied in the health care field. For further details see Warner and Luce,[3] Mills and Thomas,[4] or Drummond *et al.*[5]

EVIDENCE ON THE COSTS AND BENEFITS OF EYE HEALTH CARE

A key issue in mobilizing resources and political will is that of the relative cost effectiveness of eye health care compared to other health care interventions. Cataract operations have the advantage that they are simple, quick, and effective, and bring immediate benefits in improved quality of life. A recent study in the United

Kingdom[6] has estimated that the costs of the operation and after care in remaining years of life is around £1200 (1983 prices). By making a few additional assumptions some comparisons can be made between cataract and other health care programmes.

Williams[7] has recently reported comparisons of health care programmes in terms of their cost per QALY gained (see Table 7.1). If it is assumed that a cataract operation restores sight for the rest of the patient's life (say 10 years on average), the main unknown is the value in quality of life terms, of this improvement. There are no figures reported in the literature for the 'utility value' for cataract blindness. However, estimates are reported for renal dialysis.

Table 7.1 'League table' of costs and benefits of selected medical procedures. (Adapted from Williams 1985[7])

Procedure	Present value of extra cost per QALY gained (£)
Hip replacement	700
CABG for severe angina with left main disease	1 040
Kidney transplantation	3 000
Heart transplanation	5 000
CABG for mild angina with 2 vessel disease	12 600
Hospital haemodialysis	14 000
Cataract operation	500*

*Estimate based on Davies *et al.*[6] see text.

Therefore, if one assumed that individuals would rate cataract blindness (on a scale from 0 to 1) no better than being on renal dialysis, one might conservatively expect that restoring sight would give an improvement from 0.6 (renal dialysis) to 0.9 (nearly healthy) in cataract patients.[5] Combining the cost data with those on quality of life improvement gives a cost per QALY figure for cataract of £500 at the top of Williams' list.

Obviously this estimate needs to be treated with caution as the methodology employed here is not completely consistent with that of Williams. However, considerably more pessimistic assumptions could be made and cataract operation would still compare favourably with other investments in terms of value for money.

Unfortunately, such comprehensive data do not yet exist for developing countries. Table 7.2 shows comparative data for a range of health care programmes in terms of cost per death averted. Because cataract operation is not a life saving procedure the challenge is to develop output indices, like the QALY, for developing countries. So far the closest example to a generic outcome measure is that of 'number of healthy days of life lost' used by the Ghana Health Assessment Project Team.[8]

Table 7.2 Cost per death prevented through different health interventions

Intervention	Country	Cost per death prevented (US$)	Source
Measles immunization (includes all joint costs of a programme of polio, DPT, BCG, and tetanus)	Ivory Coast	490	Shepard (1982)
Total immunization programme	Indonesia	130	Barnum *et al.* (1980)
BCG programme only		445	
DPTT programme only		135	
BCG added to existing programme		101	
DPTT added to existing programme		77	
Mass vaccination	Morocco, 1971		Barlow (1976)
BCG		24	
DPTT		38	
Polio		1 100	
Immunization total	Kenya	85	Barnum (1980)
DPT, TT, BCG only		274	
Measles only		50	
Polio only		6 357	
DPT, TT, BCG		69	
Measles added to existing programme		26	
Polio added to existing programme		568	
New births only		70	

Table 7.2   *Continued*

			Barnum (1979)
Health programme separate	Nepal	508	
Integrated with family planning		271	
Nutrition programme prenatal	Narangwal, India	7.75	Faruqee & Johnson (1981)
Health care: infant		25	
child		31	
Hospital	Morocco, 1971		
Large		2 640	
Medium		2 820	
Small		2 360	
Hospital treatment for diarrhoea	Bangladesh	187	Horton & Claquin (1982)
Sotaki		1 262–	
Matlab		1 352	
Malaria eradication (spraying and drugs)	Bangladesh	809– 25 090	Prescott (1980)
Mosquito control—malaria (infant and child)	Cross-country analysis	600	Walsh & Warren (1979)
Community water supply, sanitation		3 600– 4 300	
Selective primary health care		200– 250	

* Adapted from Cochrane and Zachariah[10]. **For references to the individual studies see the original article.**

In one of the few economic evaluations of blindness prevention programmes in developing countries, Prost and Prescott[9] examined the cost-effectiveness of the onchocerciasis control programme in Upper Volta. They considered the number of healthy years of life added by the prevention of permanent disability and premature death attributable to onchocercal blindness. Their approach emphasized the central role of social value judgements in allocating health resources, in particular the relative weights to be assigned to preventing disability and postponing death (as discussed above).

In addition the analysis emphasized that in evaluating prevention programmes, judgements have to be made about the relative value of present and future costs and benefits. The analytical approach used to compare costs and benefits occurring at different points in time is known as *discounting to present values*. (For details see Drummond *et al.*[5]) The choice of the discount rate is a societal value judgement which may be different in different countries.

Prost and Prescott found that the cost-effectiveness estimates for blindness prevention through onchocerciasis control were US$20 per year of healthy life and per productive year of healthy life added and US$150 per discounted year of healthy life and per discounted productive year of healthy life added. They then went on to compare these estimates with those for the cost-effectiveness of measles immunization in the Ivory Coast and Zambia. They found that the relative cost-effectiveness of the different programmes was very sensitive to the choice of effectiveness measure.

In the future there are likely to be many more economic evaluations of blindness prevention programmes which will provide useful data for those arguing in support of their development. For example, an evaluation is currently underway of alternative methods to increase the uptake of cataract surgery in Southern India. An outline of the approach to economic evaluation of these options is given in the Appendix to this chapter.

OTHER ECONOMIC ISSUES

Apart from presenting economic data of the type discussed above, there are other issues that those hoping to mobilize resources for eye health care should consider. First, existing programmes should be examined to see whether they are being delivered as efficiently as possible. For example, in the case of cataract there have been initiatives to reduce the length of hospital stay, to encourage out-patient or ambulatory surgery, and to increase the use of paramedical manpower. The fact that one is continually searching for improved use of existing resources can assist one's claims for the development of programmes.

Secondly, attention needs to be paid to the incentives and disincentives operating in the health care system, to professionals, hospitals, and patients. For example, it is thought that in developing countries some individuals do not come forward for surgery because they may lose income. In addition, the methods of reimbursing hospitals and health professionals have been shown to influence their behaviour.[11] These factors need to be taken into account when developing and implementing eye health care programmes as they may have a critical impact on their cost-effectiveness.

Concluding remarks

In the future, economic data are likely to be increasingly needed in making claims for health care resources. The objective of this paper was to present some ideas that might be useful for those seeking to mobilize resources and political will in support of eye health care.

References

1. Rice, D. P. (1976). *Estimating the cost of illness*. Health Economics Series No. 6. US Public Health Service, Washington, D. C.
2. Bernth-Petersen, P. (1982). Outcome of cataract surgery. IV. Socio-economic aspects. *Acta Ophthalmologica (Copenhagen)*, **60**, 461–8.
3. Warner, K. E. and Luce, B. R. (1982). *Cost-effectiveness and cost-benefit analysis in health care: principles, practice and potential.* Health Administration Press, Ann Arbor, Michigan.
4. Mills, A. and Thomas, M. (1984). *Economic evaluation of health programmes in developing countries.* Evaluation and Planning Centre for Health Care, London School of Hygiene and Tropical Medicine, London.
5. Drummond, M. F. (1986). Financial incentives to change behaviour towards health technology. Paper prepared for the EC Workshop on Regulatory Mechanisms Concerning Expensive Health Technology, London, 22–25 April 1986.
6. Davies, L. M., Drummond, M. F., Woodward, E. G., and Buckley, R. J. (1986). A cost-effectiveness comparison of the intraocular lens and the contact lens in aphakia. *Transactions of the Ophthalmological Societies of the United Kingdom (London)*, **105**(3), 304–13.
7. Williams, A. H. (1985). Economics of coronary artery bypass grafting. *British Medical Journal (London)*, **291**, 326–9.
8. Ghana Health Assessment Project Team (1981). A quantitative method of assessing the health impact of different diseases in less developed countries. *International Journal of Epidemiology (London)*, **10**(1), 73–80.
9. Prost, A. and Prescott, N. (1984). Cost-effectiveness of blindness prevention by the onchocerciasis control programme in Upper Volta. *Bulletin of the World Health Organization (Geneva)*, **62**(5), 795–802.
10. Cochrane, S. H. and Zachariah, K. C. (1983). *Infant and child mortality as a determinant of fertility. The policy implications.* World Bank Staff Working Paper No. 556. World Bank, Washington D. C.
11. Drummond, M. F., Stoddart, G. L., and Torrance, G. W. (1986). *Methods for the economic evaluation of health care programmes.* Oxford University Press.

Appendix: Economic evaluation of methods to reduce the barriers to surgery in a developing country

One of the main problems with providing treatment for cataract in developing countries is that only a small proportion of those eligible for surgery actually have it. Although this is partly due to lack of funds and the lack of availability of ophthalmologists in some geographical locations it is also due to lack of compliance with medical advice to have surgery. Therefore, a project is currently being carried out in order to evaluate alternative approaches to overcoming the social, economic and logistic barriers to cataract surgery among rural blind individuals. Four alternatives have been identified:

(1) house-to-house visits by aphakic motivators (successfully operated cataract patients);
(2) house-to-house visits by a basic eye health worker;
(3) visits by a screening van at a central location in a village; and
(4) health education campaigns carried out at weekly marketplaces.

Under all options the cataract surgery will be carried out in the base (regional) hospital.

Each of these activities will be randomized to villages and evaluated prospectively. In addition, two different kinds of economic subsidies will be offered:

(1) free travel, food, surgery, and glasses; and
(2) free surgery and glasses only.

What steps could be taken to evaluate these options from an economic viewpoint?

Consideration of alternatives
The alternatives to be evaluated are clearly set out above. However, although it is not included in this study, the additional alternative of a mobile eye camp also merits discussion as it is the current method of choice in some locations. It might be interesting to compare the relative cost-effectiveness of these four options with the mobile eye camp, using data from earlier studies.

In addition, it should be noted that there are also alternatives in performing the cataract surgery itself, particularly the more efficient use of hospital beds, e.g. through shortening length of in-patient stay. These options may be important in reducing the over-all cost of the intervention if there are doubts about the affordability of the programme.

Assessment of effectiveness and benefit

The main measure of effectiveness in the ongoing study is the surgical coverage ratio, defined as the proportion of curable cataract blind prior to the interventions (who could benefit from surgery) who have had their sight restored within the intervention time period. Although this is entirely acceptable for a cost-effectiveness analysis, consideration could also be given to assessing the quality-adjusted life-years (QALYs) gained by the programme. This would enable comparisons to be made between this programme and those in other fields. The additional data required to estimate QALYs include the age of the patients, their likely life expectancy without cataract surgery, their vision prior to and after surgery, and the utility values of their health state prior to and after surgery. If the cataract operation were to enable any patients, or their family, to return to work there may be production benefits. However, these may be small.

Assessment of costs

The costs falling on the health sector for the given options will be those of the health workers involved, the training of these workers plus any volunteers, and supplies and items of equipment (e.g. the screening van in option 3).

If the intention in the economic evaluation was to investigate only the relative cost-effectiveness of the four ways of increasing consent to surgery, those costs which are the same for all options (e.g. the cost per patient of surgery) could be excluded. However, it would be worth-while including them if, at some later stage, the costs and benefits of this programme were to be compared with those in other fields.

Other relevant costs include those of the aphakic volunteers (in option 1) and the resource inputs from the patient and family in terms of time and expense. In principle, volunteer time should be valued in accordance with its best alternative use. It may therefore be close to zero if the volunteers merely give up leisure time to participate in the programme.

Patient and family time should also be valued in accordance with its alternative uses. These may be in work or leisure. For 50 per cent of the patients, travel and food will be paid by the health sector. Of course, this does not affect the total cost of the programme to the community as a whole, as these costs are otherwise met by the patients or their family. However, it is interesting and relevant to assess the impact of this financial incentive on the consent for surgery, even if it affects merely the relative burden of cost (between patient and health care sector), rather than the overall cost.

Allowance for differential timing of costs and benefits

Differential timing is not a major issue in this evaluation, as the time profile of costs and benefits is similar for all four alternatives. (The only exception would be equipment items, whose cost should be converted to an equivalent annual cost using a discount rate.)

Similarly, there is no reason to suppose that the estimates of cost or effectiveness are any more subject to uncertainty under one option than another. However, if estimates of cost per QALY gained were to be obtained to enable comparison with other health care programmes, a sensitivity analysis should probably be performed, investigating the impact, on cost per QALY gained, of different assumptions for some of the main variables.

8

IAPB-sponsored workshops at the Third General Assembly

GUIDELINES FOR THE TRAINING OF PARAMEDICAL
CATARACT SURGEONS

Randolph Whitfield, Jr

For more than 20 years, Ophthalmic Clinical Officers have been performing cataract surgery successfully in Kenya. Their role as cataract surgeons is not experimental but an established fact. Because of the rapidly growing backlog of patients blinded by unoperated cataract in Kenya and in other developing countries, and because of the limited resources available to train and support ophthalmologists by the governments of these countries, it appears that cataract surgery by highly trained paramedical personnel will continue to be an important strategy for the elimination of avoidable blindness in many developing countries for the foreseeable future.

Despite understandable resistance from the established medical community, over the past few years other countries have followed Kenya's lead in training non-physicians to perform cataract surgery. We can only hope that others will join them.

However, in many countries the role of the paramedical cataract surgeon remains a precarious one because there are often no accepted, standardized procedures to follow for the identification of candidates, for their training, or for their continued support and supervision in the field.

For this reason, in Kenya the National Prevention of Blindness Committee made specific recommendations to the Kenya Ministry of Health regarding:

1. the procedures for the identification of paramedical cataract surgery candidates;
2. a detailed syllabus for their surgical training; and
3. their continued supervision and support.

The following recommendations were submitted to the Kenya Ministry of Health by the Kenya National Prevention of Blindness Committee.

Cataract surgery training course for Ophthalmic Clinical Officers

This course is designed to train selected Ophthalmic Clinical Officers to become competent and safe cataract surgeons.

1. Candidates for the position of Surgical Ophthalmic Clinical Officer should be selected from those Ophthalmic Clinical Officers applying for the position who have successfully finished their training course in Ophthalmology at Kenyatta National Hospital and who have proven themselves competent and mature Ophthalmic Clinical Officers, following at least two years of satisfactory work in the field following their ophthalmic training.

2. The applications should be considered by the appropriate Provincial Ophthalmologist and those he selects for training should be approved for training by the Chief Consultant Ophthalmic Surgeon and the Director of the Ministry of Health.

3. The training period should be a minimum of 12 months, during which time the trainee should work closely with the Provincial Ophthalmologist both in his clinics and in surgery.

It is recommended that a Provincial Ophthalmologist train not more than one Ophthalmic Clinical Officer at a time, and that the training be intensive and practical in nature, providing the Clinical Officer not only with the necessary surgical expertise, but also adequate clinical ability to select suitable candidates for cataract surgery and to care for patients post-operatively.

The trainee must join his provincial Ophthalmologist at surgical sessions on a weekly basis, at a minimum; more frequently would be desirable. The candidate must become competent in the diagnosis and care of all post-operative complications.

The trainee must perform a minimum of 100 cataract extractions under supervision, and keep a careful record of the details of each case including;

    (a) indications for surgery;
    (b) a description of surgery performed including complications, if any;
    (c) post-operative course;
    (d) visual acuity and condition at discharge, and at follow up one month after surgery.

4. It is recommended that the surgical procedure taught be standardized and as simple and straightforward as possible. Although the particular training methods will vary from instructor

to instructor, every candidate must be specifically trained to become competent in the following:

(a) the diagnosis of different types of cataract, their causes, the possible complications associated with each type, and their surgical management;

(b) the indications for the need for cataract surgery for each individual presenting with the diagnosis of cataract;

(c) the complete pre-operative evaluation of each patient selected for cataract surgery, and the recognition of conditions whose presence might lead to complications during or after cataract surgery;

(d) the preparation of the patient for surgery, including:
  - discussions with the patient about what to expect before, during and after surgery, and the obtaining of legal consent from the patient, or his guardian, for the performance of the surgery;
  - the indications for and proper use of pre-operative medications, their possible complications and how to deal with them;
  - the indications for the type of cataract surgery to be performed;
  - the indications for the type of anaesthesia to be administered;
  - proper sterile operating room techniques, and sterile preparation of the patient for surgery;

(e) care of ophthalmic surgical instruments, including: proper sterilization techniques for instruments and sutures, and proper use, care, cleaning, and maintenance of ophthalmic instruments;

(f) proper administration of local anaesthesia and management of possible complications arising from their use;

(g) how to perform cataract surgery in a safe and competent manner through practical, 'hands-on', training in a one-on-one relationship with his Instructor, including:
  - extra-capsular cataract extraction;
  - intra-capsular cataract extraction;
  - needling and aspiration of cataract;
  - recognition and management of possible complications of the above surgical procedures;

(h) post-operative care of the cataract patient, including:
- the proper general care of the post-operative cataract patient, including the indications for and use of topical and systemic drugs and the recognition and treatment of the possible complications of their use;
- the ability to recognize and cope with the immediate and late complications of cataract surgery;
- post-operative counselling of the cataract patient;
- refraction and fitting of the aphakic patient with spectacles.

5. Following satisfactory completion of his course, the Candidate must then be nominated by his Instructor to become a Surgical Ophthalmic Clinical Officer.

6. This nomination must be confirmed by a second Ophthalmic Consultant after a suitable practical examination. The nomination having been confirmed, it must then be approved by the Chief Ophthalmologist and the Director of Medical Services of the Ministry of Health.

7. Supervision and support of the Surgical Ophthalmic Clinical Officer is the responsibility of the Provincial Ophthalmologist and must include regular surgical and clinical sessions together, in which pre-operative selection of surgical candidates, surgical competence, and post-operative care are constantly reassessed.

STRATEGIES TO REDUCE THE BACKLOG OF
CATARACT BLIND IN AFRICA
Randolph Whitfield, Jr.

Cataract, responsible for almost half of the blindness in the developing world, is the most pressing problem facing those concerned with avoidable blindness today.

Two factors make this immense problem even more serious. In the developing world, senile cataract affects vision at an earlier age than it does in industrialized countries. Ocular status surveys carried out in Kenya indicate that 10 per cent of those between the ages of 50 and 59 have significant visual loss from cataract, well over five times the prevalence rate of cataract affecting visual acuity in that age group in the United States.[1]

In the developing world, blindness carries with it a greatly increased mortality rate, estimated to be four times higher than for those who can see.[2]

At present, the number of cataract operations being performed in Africa, Asia, and Latin America is no where near sufficient to reduce the huge backlog of those blind from cataract, or even to keep up with the new cases occurring each year.

The question of how best to address this number one problem of blindness is a complete one, and its solution is largely determined by three major constraints that make the delivery of health care of all kinds a formidable problem:

(1) the serious shortage of trained personnel, in this case cataract surgeons;

(2) the difficulty delivering services to a population that is largely rural and often difficult to reach; and

(3) the low level of education of the majority of the people.

Manpower training

Three major strategies have been proposed to address the problem of inadequate trained manpower:

1. Train more ophthalmologists to perform cataract surgery. I estimate that there are fewer than 400 ophthalmologists at work in Africa. They are faced with 3 million cataract blind and over twice that number with significant visual loss from cataract, 9 million people needing cataract surgery. This situation is made much worse by the fact that the great majority of these eye doctors live and work in the cities, hardly ever dealing with the problems of blindness in rural areas where more than 80 per cent of the people live.

Ironically, the recent improvement in general health care, leading to greater longevity, is increasing the reservoir of people with cataract. The number of those over 50 is expected to increase by 500 per cent within the next 40 years.

In view of the training resources presently available and the tremendous need, it is clear that for the foreseeable future, ophthalmologists alone will not be able to cope with the ever-increasing backlog of cataract blind. However, the increased production of ophthalmologists will continue to be a high priority.

2. Another way to produce more cataract surgeons is the training of general physicians to perform cataract extraction. This strategy must be used most carefully. The performance of cataract extraction on a regular and frequent basis is most important to successful surgery, and the general physician or surgeon who sees but a few new cataract patients each month needing surgery is not the ideal candidate for training as a cataract surgeon.

3. A third approach to increase the number of cataract surgeons has been adopted. This is to train paramedical eye workers to perform cataract extraction. The advantages of training eye auxiliaries to work in the place of ophthalmologists are obvious and significant. More can be trained in a shorter time and at less cost; their continued support costs are considerably less; their surgical results are excellent; and they are more willing to work in rural areas than ophthalmologists.

Important to their success as cataract surgeons is the great frequency with which they perform the operation. Studies carried out by me and by others have demonstrated conclusively that the many thousands of blind people who have had their sight restored by paramedical cataract surgeons have not received second-rate ophthalmic care. Eye auxiliaries make excellent cataract surgeons and their surgical results have been demonstrated to be comparable to those obtained by ophthalmologists.[3]

In view of the immense need for cataract surgeons, and the demonstrated ability of paramedical surgeons to perform cataract extraction in a highly capable and professional manner, this is a most valuable strategy. Ophthalmologists are such an invaluable and rare resource that they must be utilized as efficiently as possible, and their work must be limited to that which cannot be carried out by others.

Means to improve the efficiency of providing cataract surgery

The problem of efficiently reaching a largely rural population has been approached in several different ways.

In India the cataract camp has proven to be an invaluable strategy. In its most highly developed form, cataract camps have restored sight to 5 million Indians during the last five years, through the provision of cataract surgery of the highest quality.

However, in Africa cataract camps have not proven to be of much value. There they are expensive, with the cost per operation typically several times the cost of routine hospital surgery; the number of patients coming to cataract camps has been small despite extensive promotional activity; pre-operative evaluation and post-operative follow-up have been poor; and the visual results of camp surgery have often been disappointing compared to the results of routine cataract extractions performed in a hospital setting.

Another suggestion to improve the efficiency of cataract surgery has been to decrease the period of post-operative hospitalization. In Africa, because of the typical conditions at home to which a rural patient is discharged, the in-hospital post-operative period of five days cannot be safely shortened.

Another suggestion has been to perform cataract surgery on an out-patient basis. Although over 90 per cent of all cataract surgery in the United States is performed as an out-patient procedure, this is not a viable strategy for Africa. Not only is it medically unwise to discharge patients immediately following surgery, but it makes no sense whatsoever from an economic point of view. The single most important cost in providing cataract surgery to rural Africans is the cost of transportation. To consider the prospect of multiple trips to and from the surgical facility for follow-up is totally unrealistic.

In Africa, mobile eye units have been used for many years to bring eye care services to the people. Although the capital and running costs of mobile eye unit programmes have increased dramatically during the past several years, there will continue to be a need for such services in many outlying and underserved areas for decades to come.

However, in many areas the population density is increasing, and public transport is improving dramatically. In these areas it has become more cost-effective to train ophthalmic paramedical workers and provide simple outlying static eye clinics for them to work in. Static clinics have the additional real benefit of providing the residents of the surrounding areas with year-round, rather than intermittent, eye care services.

The role of health education

The final major constraint in addressing the problem of cataract blind in Africa is the lack of awareness, particularly among the rural majority, that cataract blindness can be cured by a safe and relatively simple operation.

A major problem is that many blinded by cataract simply are not aware that their vision can be restored. In Kenya, where we have a huge and growing number of people needing cataract surgery, I estimate that less than 3000 cataract extractions are performed annually, yet few of our eye departments have large backlogs of patients waiting for a cataract operation.

A recent ocular status survey in a Middle-Eastern country having one of the highest per capita incomes in the world revealed a prevalence of blindness of 1.5 per cent. Unoperated cataract accounted for 55 per cent of this blindness. This clearly illustrates that people must be informed about the causes of blindness, and motivated to take the necessary action.

Thus, to address effectively the backlog of cataract blind, health educational activities designed to inform the people of the safety, value, and availability of cataract surgery must receive the highest priority.

In summary, I have briefly discussed some of the major problems involved in addressing cataract blindness in Africa, and some of the strategies that have been developed to solve them. Foremost among these problems are: the lack of trained cataract surgeons, the difficulties in providing services to the rural poor, and the lack of awareness among the rural poor that cataract extraction is a safe and effective cure for cataract blindness. In Africa, strategies to address these problems include: the training of more ophthalmologists; the training and utilization of paramedical cataract surgeons; both mobile and static eye care delivery systems, depending upon the local situation; and effective health education.

References

1. Podgor, M. J., Leske, C. L., and Ederer, F. (1983). Incidence estimates for lens changes, macular changes, open-angle glaucoma and diabetic retinopathy. *American Journal of Epidemiology (Baltimore)*, **118**, 206.
2. Prost, A. and Paris, F. (1983). L'incidence de la cécité et ses aspects epidemiologiques dans une region rurale de l'Afrique de l'Ouest. *WHO Bulletin*, **61**(2), 491–99.
3. Whitfield, R. (1984). Kenya rural blindness prevention project. In *World blindness and its prevention*, Vol. 2 (ed. IAPB), pp. 69–74. Oxford University Press.

MULTI-DISCIPLINARY APPROACHES TO CHILDREN AND CORNEAL DISEASE

Barbara A. Underwood

Corneal disease due to keratomalacia, or secondary to trauma, is the major cause of preventable blindness among children. It is a problem that for prevention and treatment requires the combined attention of the health care system and other sectors that influence community awareness, education and practices.

Prevention of corneal disease and preventable blindness requires that health workers increase their understanding and awareness of the problem and appropriate solutions. They are the primary contact point for diagnosis of disease and immediate treatment as well as respected advisers for prevention. Materials have been developed by the World Health Organization (WHO), and others, for training all levels of the health system in recognizing corneal disease, its causes, and appropriate curative or preventive measures. Greater efforts are needed to enhance the incorporation of these materials into training programmes of primary eye and health care workers and professionals at the secondary level.

Keratomalacia as a cause of childhood blindness is an avertable tragedy. Treatment necessitates a medical approach; its long-term prevention necessitates non-medical interventions. It is due to a dietary deficiency of vitamin A commonly associated also with a dietary deficit of protein and energy. Although family economics is a factor, poor child-feeding practices are most often the cause of an inadequate diet. National prevention programmes, which provide coverage of the preschool population with a periodic high-dose supplement of vitamin A, are effective in preventing blindness, but in the case of keratomalacia address only one component of the dietary deficiency problem. In addition, the incomplete coverage these programmes suffer from frequently miss those children who are most malnourished and at greatest risk. Furthermore, such programmes are difficult to sustain. Although theoretically capable of high coverage, approaches through fortification of a common food vehicle have not yet proven to be sustainable in non-industrialized countries. More importantly, neither of these short-term interventions address the underlying issue of inadequate child-feeding practices. Behavioural changes within families are required to achieve long-term, sustainable prevention.

Greater awareness of, access of, and utilization in children's diets of vitamin A-rich food sources locally available and culturally acceptable could permanently avert much of the keratomalacia problem. However, health and nutrition education programmes developed and implemented vertically by the health sector have been notoriously ineffective. Increasingly, it is being recognized that developing appropriate programmes and effectively communicating these require multi-faceted horizontal actions. A key to producing effective educational materials and programmes has been to adapt solutions to those applicable locally and presenting these within the local, culturally appropriate context. Some examples include home or kitchen gardening approaches that are jointly designed and implemented by horticulturalists working with anthropologists to maximally utilize limited space and inputs to gain maximum outputs of vitamin A-rich foods that young children will eat.

Some innovative programmes are underway in which health and nutrition education personnel are combining efforts with those versed in communication. Advanced communication techniques are being used as are traditional arts, which are being targeted toward prevention, for example changes in behaviours. In some areas, social marketing techniques, using the mass media, have effectively increased awareness of the problem and are now being evaluated for their long-term influence in changing dietary behaviour patterns. In parts of Asia among more traditional societies, approaches using folk arts to communicate messages of health education, safety, and nutrition have been well received and effective in achieving behavioural changes in the short run. Their effectiveness in sustained behaviour change is being monitored in some programmes.

PREVENTION AND REHABILITATION: THEIR COMPLEMENTARY RELATIONSHIP IN NATIONAL PROGRAMMES

Sally Deitz and *Eva Friedlander*

The workshop on prevention and rehabilitation introduced the issue of rehabilitation into an I A PB General Assembly for the first time. It was opened by Sir John Wilson, who stated that his intention was that the audience participate in this panel, that each panelist give a brief presentation and then the floor would be turned over to those present. The panelists included Dr Sally Deitz, Mr Samir Jain, Dr G. Kothari, and Dr V. S. Chandraseka.

Dr Deitz's introductory statement, prepared with Dr Friedlander, also of the American Foundation for the Blind, and Larry Campbell of Helen Keller International, set the framework for the session as a whole. An overview of some of the major issues in designing rehabilitation internationally was presented as were policy considerations for the future.

First, the importance of considering the socio-cultural context in which rehabilitation takes place was addressed, and in particular the nature of those services and the location of their provision. The panelists emphasized that amidst all the statistics and demographic data on the number of cataract surgeries, number of trachoma cases, etc. it is essential to remember that behind every eye there is a person, and behind every person, a family, a community, and an entire social structure in which the services are embedded and upon which their success depends. These structures, such as the extended family, can be used effectively to develop rehabilitation services. Rehabilitation is, therefore, best offered closest to the space and time in which the visually handicapped will use the skills they are being taught. Those who are part of the culture, speak the language, and know its resources are the appropriate people to design and offer the services. In addition, there is the danger of introducing a rehabilitation structure designed on a conventional US model that may, as described by Robert Scott in *The making of blind men*, further disable—rather than help—visually impaired clients in terms of economics, employment, and socialization.

The essential components of effective rehabilitation programmes were outlined. They include: (1) teaching critical, functional skills needed and used in the homes and workplaces; (2) teaching in the natural environment in which the skills are to be used, most often the village or community in which the person lives; (3) assuring that the skills taught are culturally and age-appropriate; (4) aiming at normalization of access, with the goal of providing disabled persons with equal access to vocational, social, and economic choices to those of able-bodied persons in that culture; and (5) emphasis on the strengths and capabilities of the individuals, rather than the pathology of the disability.

It was pointed out that in contrast to conventional formal rehabilitation, community-based rehabilitation is 35 to 60 per cent less expensive per capita. Cost alone, however, is only one of the many reasons why community-based rehabilitation is becoming recognized as the preferred practice.

Planning

The importance of making rehabilitation a priority for the future was raised. It entails the need to focus on two levels: first, the policy-making and legislative level and second, the grassroots level. At the policy and planning level the education of government leaders and education and rehabilitation administrators was described as critical for change. Equally critical is the involvement of visually impaired consumers as advocates and as participants at all stages of policy making and programme planning, both in governmental and non-governmental organizations such as IAPB.

At the grassroots level the need to increase public awareness, communicate the need for services, and integrate programmes suitable to the population was touched upon. The need for coalitions with other disability groups was stressed as a way to strengthen recognition and effect change at both levels.

Finally, work for the disabled has traditionally been seen as charitable, entailing a patronizing attitude that is often far more disabling than the absence of conventional services. People need to be encouraged to view such services as a *right*, rather than a gift.

In closing, three beginning steps were suggested for planning a national programme and developing partnerships between prevention and rehabilitation: (1) to include visually impaired people in planning at every level both in prevention and rehabilitation; (2) to begin dialogues among people in medical care, education, and rehabilitation of the visually handicapped; and (3) to view critically the established services already in place and address questions regarding the efficacy of those services and their role in creating lives of dignity and participation for the visually handicapped persons they seek to serve.

During the very wide-ranging discussion that followed the panel presentations, the audience provided a highly varied perspective on the issues raised. Some of the most striking contributions included: (1) a criticism of an approach that emphasizes cost-effectiveness; (2) the perception that blind persons are distanced by language that suggests 'us versus them'; and (3) the possible philosophical contradictions underlying the approaches of prevention and rehabilitation.

In conclusion, Sir John Wilson stated optimistically that IAPB wished to continue to bridge the gap between prevention and rehabilitation. He pledged the support of IAPB in this effort and said that he looked forward to continuing the discussion of these issues at future IAPB General Assemblies.

9

Recommendations of the Executive Board accepted by the General Assembly

The following resolutions were drafted and unanimously approved by the Executive Board at their meeting on 7 and 8 December 1986. They were unanimously accepted by the General Assembly at the Concluding Plenary Session on 10 December 1986.

REGIONS, REGIONAL CHAIRMEN, BUDGETS, AND MEMBERSHIP

1. IAPB regions should be co-terminus with those of the World Health Organization, allowing for the establishment of appropriate subdivisions within each region.

2. Duties of a Regional or Subregional Chairman should include: effective and continuous contact with all national committees in the region; assistance in strengthening existing committees and, where necessary, initiating new committees; overseeing the organization, where practical, of regional or subregional conferences; and acting as the Agency's link with Regional Committees of the World Health Organization, and with the regional structures of the International Federation of Ophthalmological Societies, the World Blind Union, and IAPB's international member organizations.

3. A central budget should be formulated, that international non-governmental organizations and other appropriate organizations and individuals should be requested to make financial commitments to support that budget over the next several years and that a subcommittee of the Executive Board, called the Executive Committee, should meet and discuss options for funding the Agency's activities.

4. A system of membership and subscription should be established that will identify all categories of members, including life membership within the Agency, and that will enable each region to set and collect its own subscriptions with, where appropriate, separate rates for organizations and individuals within each region or subregion and that will ensure that all members receive information, including the

Agency's newsletter, from the central headquarters of the Agency.

5. Each regional Chairman or Chairmen should, therefore, formulate a regional budget and take action to raise the necessary funds within each region, possibly by establishing regional foundations with fund-raising capacity. It is understood that the relatively small amounts involved at the regional level would not constitute serious competition with the fund-raising activities of the international Non-governmental Organization.

CATARACT BACKLOG

The Third General Assembly of IAPB is concerned about the great backlog of unoperated cataract in many developing countries and recommends that:

6. Increased resources should be mobilized and made available by governments, non-governmental organizations, ophthalmic societies, and all other possible groups or individuals, for the elimination of the cataract backlog in the countries concerned.

7. Specifically, more manpower should be made available for cataract surgery through: increased teaching of cataract surgeons and increased cataract surgery by existing surgeons, with particular involvement of the ophthalmic professionals not yet active in this field.

8. Research and practical trials should be conducted to optimize the management and procedures for increased numbers of cataract operations in existing eye departments.

9. Increased attention should be paid to reducing the period of hospitalization for cataract surgery; this is possible using an improved surgical technique for wound closure, and provided measures are taken to ensure patient compliance and availability for post-operative care.

10. Careful monitoring and evaluation should be included as part of the action taken to reduce the cataract backlog, to allow for an assessment of the progress made in the countries concerned.

10

International non-governmental organizations

COMMUNICATIONS BETWEEN NON-GOVERNMENTAL
ORGANIZATIONS AND THE WORLD HEALTH
ORGANIZATION

Bjorn Thylefors

The important role of non-governmental organizations (NGOs)
working in the field of health has been recognized by the World
Health Organization (WHO) since its inception. Rules and criteria
have, for a long time, been laid down for collaboration between
NGOs and WHO, leading to the concept of 'official relations', in
which there is an officially recognized area of co-operation, and a
workplan. This co-operation is reviewed periodically at three-year
intervals, and there are at present some 155 NGOs in official working relations with WHO, representing a wide variety of health care
fields.

The main components of collaboration at the global level between
NGOs and WHO are usually the exchange of information between
the organizations, attendance at each other's meetings, and periodic
reporting or consultations. There are also joint activities involving
training courses or provision of learning materials for health personnel of all categories, and data collection for setting of standards and
development of guidelines. The World Health Assembly in 1985
considered in its Technical Discussions collaboration with non-
governmental organizations for the attainment of 'Health for All by
the Year 2000', and this has been an important step in the further
strengthening of co-operation.

The WHO Programme for the Prevention of Blindness collaborates closely with several NGOs, particularly as part of its collaboration with the International Agency for the Prevention of
Blindness (IAPB). In fact, IAPB was involved in the early stage of
launching the WHO Programme, playing the role of an 'umbrella
organization' for several NGOs in relation to WHO. The WHO

Programme for the Prevention of Blindness has since become one of the leading programmes in terms of collaboration with NGOs, and the example is now being followed by other WHO health programmes.

The communication channels at the global level are mainly:

(1) participation of interested NGOs in the meetings of the WHO Programme Advisory Group on the Prevention of Blindness;

(2) exchange of information material, reports, etc.;

(3) informal consultations, as needed with each NGO; and

(4) consultations through the new Consultative Group of NGOs to the WHO Programme, established in 1986. This group meets at least at yearly intervals.

Whereas communications and co-operation are generally successful at the global level, much remains to be done at the regional and national levels. Following the Technical Discussions at the World Health Assembly in 1985, some of the WHO Regional Committees are addressing the issue of strengthening collaboration with NGOs. At the national level, the national committees for the prevention of blindness have proved to be a very useful forum for bringing together national authorities, NGOs, and others interested in blindness prevention.

There are several points that have been of particular importance in contributing to the development of a fruitful collaboration between WHO and NGOs in the field of blindness prevention. The joint development of the primary health care approach to the prevention of blindness, including the promotion of primary eye care, has no doubt been of importance, as this has also laid the basis for work with national authorities. The close communication between NGOs and WHO in the promotion and dissemination of information on blindness prevention, as well as the opportunities for easy mutual consultations have certainly been other important factors facilitating the development of collaborative activities.

REPORTS OF THE NON-GOVERNMENTAL
ORGANIZATIONS

The following non-governmental organizations (NGOs) make significant contributions to regional and national prevention of blindness programmes, and are affiliated with the IAPB. They work closely with the WHO Programme Advisory Group on the

Prevention of Blindness, government agencies, other voluntary organizations, and with each other.

Christoffel-Blindenmission

The Christoffel-Blindenmission (CBM), a non-governmental international organization was founded nearly 80 years ago. It is based in Bensheim, Federal Republic of Germany. CBM is and has been committed to establishing medical and rehabilitation programmes for the blind, visually impaired, and physically handicapped persons on four continents.

Named in honour of Pastor Ernst Christoffel, who worked from 1908 to 1955 among blind and handicapped people in the Middle East, CBM has grown rapidly in the past 25 years and is now reaching out to 95 countries in Asia, Africa, Latin America, and Oceania. Regional offices have been established in Malaysia, Thailand, India, Kenya, Togo, the Dominican Republic, and Paraguay. These offices have engaged the services of expert personnel in the fields of ophthalmology, optometry, education, and rehabilitation who guide, counsel, and advise headquarters in all decision-making processes.

In contrast with other similar organizations, CBM has refrained from establishing and implementing its own projects overseas. Instead, CBM supports national activities of missions, churches, and voluntary agencies in developing countries. The support is manifold: financial aid to cover operational expenses, provision of equipment, drugs, medicines, and instruments: but even more importantly, the secondment of expert personnel (at present 203 co-workers), who help to plan and carry out programmes for those who are sick and disabled.

In 1986 alone, treatment was given to over 2 million patients and this included a total of over 180 000 operations of which 110 000 were for cataract. CBM has recently pioneered the mass production of simple spectacles by appropriate methods and in 1986 distributed more than 250 000 glasses. In addition, 660 000 schoolchildren were screened and support was given to 234 schools for the disabled with a total of more than 19 000 pupils.

It is self-evident that the battle against world blindness cannot be fought with traditional ophthalmology and rehabilitation alone. The prevention of blindness requires a multi-disciplinary effort involving the ophthalmologist for treatment; the optometrist for application of special aids; the health worker to assist the family; the vocational rehabilitation counsellor to evaluate skills and to plan placement, self-employment, and workshop programmes; and a corps of community volunteers to co-ordinate and stimulate project participation.

The required funds of CBM's extensive services are raised entirely from hundreds of thousands of individual donors in Germany and some other European countries. In recent years affiliates known as 'Christian Blind Mission International' were established in the United States, Canada, and Australia to motivate more donors in those parts of the world. Roughly 50 per cent of last year's annual income of DM88 million was sent for medical/ophthalmic programmes, whereas the other half was distributed among partners catering to the educational and rehabilitational needs of disabled people and, in particular, those who are blind.

While assisting in 920 overseas projects at the grassroots level, CBM also contributes to international efforts in the battle against blindness. CBM has made contributions to research on onchocerciasis, xerophthalmia, and glaucoma. CBM has also helped to establish the International Agency for the Prevention of Blindness (in partnership with the Royal Commonwealth Society for the Blind), and co-operates with internationally recognized organizations.

Further information from: Christoffel-Blindenmission, Nibelungenstrasse 124, D-6140 Bensheim 4, Federal Republic of Germany.

Foresight

Foresight is the only international non-government organization in Australia supported by charitable donations. It is concerned solely with overseas prevention and alleviation of blindness. The origins of Foresight began in 1978 within the Australian National Council of and for the Blind. It is now a fully incorporated independent organization but retains representatives from the ANCB and other community groups on its Board.

Foresight activities now extend into many developing countries and its activities are increasing as a result of it becoming a member of the partnership arrangement with the Royal Commonwealth Society for the Blind, Helen Keller International, Operation Eyesight Universal, and the International Eye Foundation.

Current programmes of Foresight include:

Bangladesh Since 1928, Foresight with the Royal Commonwealth Society for the Blind has been responsible for training of eye health personnel, including doctors and Paramedics in Bangladesh, at the Chittagong Eye Infirmary and Training Complex. The programme is an incountry training programme based at the Chittagong Eye Infirmary and Training Complex. Doctors and paramedics trained now serve in eight base hospitals throughout Bangladesh.

In 1983 Foresight shared with the Royal Commonwealth Society for the Blind in the building of the training complex. Contributions to the hospital were made largely through the co-operation of Andheri Hilfe, together with the governments of the United Kingdom, West Germany, and Australia.

In 1983, Foresight established the clinical microbiology services at the Chittagong Eye Infirmary and Training Complex (CEITC), and trained the paramedical and medical personnel to run it. In addition, a number of eye health personnel have been identified and trained; and given opportunity for a further work experience and qualifications in Australia. These personnel have been in the areas of theatre sterilization and administration, ward administration, and clinical microbiology.

A Diploma of Community Ophthalmology has been established in the University of Chittagong, currently a Chair and a Department of Community Ophthalmology is being endowed. The Staff will be sited at the CEITC, which will ultimately provide the expertise and leadership to run the programme of teaching and eye health services at the level of primary, secondary and tertiary care for the Chittagong area, urban and rural.

Western Samoa   Equipment and training of ophthalmology and development of spectacle services.

Fiji   Low vision services. Currently a survey into the causes of blindness in the Fiji School for the Blind is being conducted.

China   Low vision training in Australia, and an exchange of personnel for work experience with Beijing and the Tianjin University.

Papua New Guinea   Support of development of eye departments and eye care centres. Vision care and training, and assistance with Braille production.

India   Training Low Vision Manager for the Low Vision Centre in Bombay.

Nepal   Equipment for operating on congenital cataract. These services are in addition to the exchange of personnel with Thailand, China, and Tonga. Furthermore Foresight is involved in provision of library materials in Braille (Bangladesh, India, Sri Lanka, China, and Papua New Guinea).

Further information from: The Secretary, Foresight, PO Box 162, Kew, Victoria, 3101, Australia.

Helen Keller International

Helen Keller International (HKI) advances indigenous capacities to prevent blindness in nations where untreated eye disease is a problem of public health proportion. Special attention is given to increasing the access of rural peoples to primary eye care, to the control of xerophthalmia, and to the restoration of sight for cataract victims. The agency also responds to emergency situations, like the African drought, which put huge numbers of people at severely increased risk of blindness. For the irrevocably blind, HKI establishes community-based rehabilitation services and trains teachers to receive blind children in existing village classrooms.

HKI aims to establish low-cost community-based care that can be sustained with local resources after HKI consultants depart. A pre-condition of assistance is the existence of at least a skeleton health care network and, where possible, HKI joins forces with supranational agencies and other non-governmental organizations engaged in fostering health and development. Typically, HKI begins with geographically limited programmes in which methods for surveying disease prevalence, training personnel, delivering care, and evaluating effects can be tested quickly and replicated easily. Operations research is conducted to assure the efficiency of the interventions.

HKI turned to the prevention of xerophthalmia in the early-1970s, with work that established the magnitude of the disease and an immediate solution: biannual megadoses of 200 000 iu of vitamin A administered orally to malnourished children under the age of six. Since that time, HKI has assisted the governments of Indonesia, Bangladesh, and the Philippines in Asia, and El Salvador and Haiti in Latin America, among others, to launch a variety of programmes that will save small children from the consequences of vitamin A deficiency. More recently, the African nations of Burkina Faso, Ethiopia, Malawi, Mali, Mauritania, Niger, and Sudan have joined the list. An added impetus to this work comes from studies of the mid-1980s, carried out with the collaboration of HKI, which show that children who are deficient in vitamin A are not only subject to ocular disease, but also die at a significantly higher rate than children with adequate stores of vitamin A.

To meet both ongoing and emergency needs for vitamin A among children of many nations, HKI has developed a number of strategies, including distribution of megadose capsules, nutrition education, and encouragement of home gardens containing dark green leafy vegetables. Studies to determine the efficiency of alternate delivery systems for the vitamin A (for example, capsule versus liquid dispenser, house-to-house distribution versus central sites), aim to bring costs down while maintaining or increasing effectiveness. Long-term solutions being explored and attempted under the aegis of HKI are food fortification, 'social marketing' to change dietary behaviour, and computer databanks that will sift through existing health records to uncover regions with vitamin A deficient children.

Primary eye care programmes in Peru, the Philippines, Sri Lanka, Indonesia, Fiji, Papua New Guinea, Solomon Islands, Tanzania, and Morocco train and equip a range of health workers to integrate an eye care component into the basic health care generally available at the community level. Trachoma is singled out for special attention where it is endemic; and in Tanzania, HKI is taking part in a long-term study of trachoma risk factors and intervention strategies. In each country, cases requiring the attention of an ophthalmologist, most often for cataract extraction, are referred to district or regional hospitals newly staffed and supplied for eye surgery with HKI assistance.

HKI also mounts projects directed specifically at reducing the backlog of unoperated cataract patients. Among these are the creation of 'cataract-free' zones in Latin America, by means of crash programmes to treat most persons blind from bilateral cataracts within a short time; identification of cataract-blind in Bali and in Shun-Yi County, China, and motivating them to surgery; furnishing mobile clinics to bring surgical services to rural areas outside of Canton; training medical assistants to perform cataract surgery in Malawi; and, in India, enabling a leading eye clinic to establish a programme to teach efficient hospital management to administrators and physicians.

When HKI was founded by Helen Keller and other Americans in 1915, it was for the express purpose of helping to rehabilitate blind persons outside the United States. That mission continues today in many developing countries with the agency's programmes to train local field workers, usually young adults, to impart to their blind clients skills for daily living and for a village-based trade. The goal is to make blind persons self-sufficient quickly and inexpensively. Blind babies receive special attention in HKI projects that teach parents to compensate for a lack of sight during the infant–toddler period of learning, and to prepare the child for formal schooling. The next step, ideally, is 'integrated education', another programme pioneered by HKI, whereby teachers of sighted children are enabled to instruct students who are dependent on braille materials or who need special attention because of low vision.

HKI publishes training materials, manuals, conference proceedings, assessments of blindness, and other technical works that are useful to the world community of workers in blindness prevention.

Further information from: Helen Keller International Inc. 15 West 16th Street, New York, NY 10011, USA.

International Eye Foundation

For the past 25 years the International Eye Foundation (IEF) has been providing humanitarian and development assistance to the developing world based upon a philosophy of helping others to help themselves. At the request of governments, the IEF provides technical assistance in determining the cause, extent, and resources available to treat blinding eye disease, and designs integrated programmes appropriate to the needs and resources of the country.

Caribbean   Since 1983, the International Eye Foundation has been involved in a collaborative effort to establish a course of study for general practitioners from the Caribbean leading to a Diploma in Ophthalmology at the Barbados campus of the University of West Indies. Physicians from Dominica, Grenada, St. Lucia, St. Vincent, Belize, and Barbados who have been trained through this programme now provide qualified, regular eye care to their home islands where ophthalmic services were previously unavailable.

The IEF has also provided ophthalmic training to nurses working in relatively isolated island communities in hospital settings and among district nurses, family nurse practitioners and community health workers located in rural areas.

The IEF continues its programme of service and training on the islands of Grenada and St. Lucia, the latter in collaboration with Massachusetts Eye and Ear Infirmary. Approximately 20 000 patients a year are seen and over 400 major surgeries performed on these two islands alone. In 1985, the IEF also assumed responsibility for providing eye care on the islands of St. Kitts and Nevis.

In 1986, in collaboration with Howard University, Washington, D.C., the IEF undertook a glaucoma survey on the island of St. Lucia.

Dominican Republic   A two year primary eye care project in the Dominican Republic was completed in September 1985. This project involved several components: training various levels of health personnel and community educators, providing basic ophthalmic equipment to central hospitals, providing appropriate ophthalmic aides to regional health centres, and organizing specialized teaching conferences for the national ophthalmological society. Through this project, over 500 general physicians, 80 registered nurses, 380 auxiliary nurses, and 5900 health promoters were taught the basics of primary eye care.

Egypt   In 1984, the Society of Eye Surgeons, the medical arm of the I E F, held its Fifth World Congress in Cairo. Over 1000 ophthalmologists from around the world participated. The theme of the conference was ophthalmology and blindness prevention in the developing world.

In 1985, a two-year project, centered in a poor section of Cairo, was completed. Over 600 health workers received training in primary eye care and blindness prevention. Two ocular surveys were also undertaken in co-operation with the Egyptian Nutrition Institute to determine the prevalence and etiology of blindness in rural and urban areas. Over one million dollars worth of supplies and equipment were provided to the Ministry of Health for use in its ophthalmic programmes.

Guinea   A new national ophthalmic referral centre based in the capital, Conakry, was refurbished and equipped by the I E F.

Kenya   In 1984, I E F's Kenya Rural Blindness Prevention Project was completed. Several hundred health workers received training in primary eye care and blindness prevention, which enabled them to provide essential eye care services in areas previously without regular eye care.

Since then, the I E F has continued to supervise the Primary Eye Care and Blindness Prevention Education Unit of the Ministry of Health. During 1984 and 1985, over 2000 health workers and primary school teachers received training through this unit. The Ministry of Health's training programme for ophthalmic clinical officers was also reorganized under I E F auspices.

Puerto Rico   Since 1968, the I E F has provided fellowships to over 500 Latin American physicians to undertake training in the basic science course in ophthalmology at the University of Puerto Rico.

Honduras   In 1983, the IEF completed a three-year programme in which over 1250 health care workers received training in blindness prevention and primary eye care. Since 1983, the IEF has continued to provide training, both in primary eye care and in more technically sophisticated areas such as retinal and corneal disease. In 1985, a laser was provided to San Felipe Hospital and a group of ophthalmologists trained in its use. A new three-year training programme based in San Pedro Sula began in 1986. This new project will train community health promoters in rural areas in primary eye care and develop the capacity of the referral hospital to handle a growing patient load.

Ecuador   An eye care project is beginning in Ecuador where rural physicians and nurses will be trained in primary eye care and rural screening programmes developed. Training will be provided not only to Ministry of Health personnel but also to health workers active in private voluntary organizations.

Saudi Arabia   In 1983, the IEF conducted a major study of blindness and eye disease in conjunction with the Ministry of Health and King Khaled Eye Specialist Hospital. During the course of the survey nearly 17 000 individuals throughout the country were examined. Results from this survey have subsequently been published.

Malawi   In 1983, the first class of ophthalmic medical assistants graduated from the Southern African Sub-regional Ophthalmic Training Centre which emerged as a result of successful interagency co-operation including IEF, the Royal Commonwealth Society for the Blind, WHO, Operation Eyesight Universal, and the government of Malawi. Graduates of this course have been drawn from Malawi, Swaziland, Botswana, Lesotho, Zambia, and Zimbabwe.

In 1983, the IEF also undertook a major study of nutritional eye disease in children and blindness prevalence in Malawi's Lower Shire Valley in collaboration with other agencies. During a three-month survey, over 7000 people were given complete ocular examinations and 5000 children were examined for nutritional deficiencies.

A major new programme was launched in the Lower Shire Valley in 1985 to reduce childhood mortality and blindness and visual loss. The project will promote the use of oral rehydration therapy and expand the Ministry of Health's current immunization programmes in addition to undertaking more specific blindness prevention activities.

Ethiopia One major outcome of the drought and famine in Ethiopia has been a substantial increase in the prevalence of blindness and visual impairment caused by nutritional deficiencies. To meet the need for the establishment of an effective eye health care system, the IEF plans to assist the Government in the development of ophthalmic manpower at the secondary level. The IEF in collaboration with Helen Keller International, the Ministry of Health, and the faculty of medicine at Addis Ababa University will establish a one-year training programme to provide the Ministry of Health with primary eye care workers to work in unserved rural areas.

Zimbabwe In 1986, IEF began a three-year project to assist the Ministry of Health in the development of an appropriate eye health care system. Specifically, the project will train ophthalmic medical assistants at the central, provincial, and district levels and train general health workers in the provision of primary eye care at the rural and village levels. Training capabilities at the central and provincial hospital level will also be upgraded.

Further information from: International Eye Foundation, 7801 Norfolk Avenue, Bethesda, Maryland 20814, USA.

Operation Eyesight Universal

Operation Eyesight Universal (OEU) was founded in Calgary, Canada in 1963. It funds sight restoration and blindness prevention programmes in 14 countries of the developing world. Seventy-six teams of Nationals are in the programme today.

It all started when a Canadian medical missionary, Dr Ben Gullison, went to India in 1933 with his bride. They settled in Sompeta on the east coast in an area in which lived 200 000 curable blind people. Dr Gullison returned to Canada in the winter of 1962/63 and tried to stimulate Canadians to assist him in the financing of his programme. In the large audience in Calgary a handful of businessmen heard his message and several months later started Operation Eyesight Universal. In 1963, 148 blind persons were restored to sight. In 1985, OEU teams treated 1 203 372 people and gave sight to 92 184 individuals.

The projects assisted through Operation Eyesight Universal include eye hospitals, eye departments in general hospitals, eye clinics, mobile eye units, and training of personnel at all levels from primary health care personnel to ophthalmologists.

Further information from: Operation Eyesight Universal, PO Box 123, Station 'M', Calgary, Alberta T2P 2H6, Canada.

Royal Commonwealth Society for the Blind

The Royal Commonwealth Society for the Blind (RCSB) was founded in 1950 on the initiative of British and Commonwealth Governments and with the active co-operation of national organizations for the blind. The Society is based in the United Kingdom but administers its programmes through regional offices in India, Bangladesh, Kenya, and Malaysia, and directly through the Caribbean Council for the Blind in that region. These offices work in liaison with national partner organizations in the 32 Commonwealth countries in which the Society operates. RCSB presently disburses just under US$6 million per annum: 50 per cent of this is accounted for by programming in Asia, 35 per cent in Africa, and the remainder in the Caribbean, Oceania, and in Inter-Commonwealth programmes. These monies are raised from a number of non-government sources in the United Kingdom, from co-financing arrangements with partner international organizations and from government matching grants.

RCSB's work initially revolved around the provision of education and rehabilitation to the incurably blind. While this work continues, and today accounts for just over 30 per cent of the annual overseas expenditure, the Society has increasingly become involved in the provision of preventative and curative eye care which utilizes the balance of its budget. Beginning in the 1960s, with mobile eye unit programmes in Africa, the Society extended its activities to South Asia where it pioneered the massive eye camp programme that presently seeks to reduce the cataract backlog in the Subcontinent. Currently, the Society supports over 200 000 cataract operations annually at hundreds of camps throughout India and Bangladesh. In addition, in India, the Society is funding a large-scale attack on the scourge of nutritional blindness in young children through its Xerophthalmia Programme. The Society's present policy in Asia is to continue to support eye camps but also to support the construction and running of small rural hospitals as a year-round solution to the cataract and general eye care problems for all age groups. Meanwhile, in Africa, the mobile eye unit programme, serving millions of people living in inaccessible rural areas, has continued to expand. RCSB presently funds the operations of 50 mobile eye units working in 11 Commonwealth African countries.

In recognition of the acute shortage of skilled ophthalmic personnel at all levels, the Society is heavily involved in manpower development through sponsorship of courses in community ophthalmology in Britain and in Asia and the direct funding of training courses for ophthalmic clinical assistants in Malawi, Kenya, Tanzania, and Bangladesh. When trained, such staff become an integral part of the eye care provision network, working at the primary level with mobile eye units and in rural based hospitals, providing primary eye care education, treating simple cases, and diagnosing and referring more complex cases to secondary and tertiary facilities.

RCSB's continuing education and rehabilitation programming focuses on the integration of the incurably blind into community life. In education, this is attained through the promotion of primary schooling in normal schools, using itinerant specialist teachers and providing basic braille equipment, of which the Society has distributed over 12 000 kits to date. In rehabilitation, the Society is funding field-based rural rehabilitation programmes throughout the Commonwealth. These vary in their specific characteristics but all are aimed at training blind people in basic living skills, and where possible, in income generating rural skills, in the blind person's own environment as an alternative to institutional provision.

Through working on priority projects in some of the poorest communities in the world, the Society has already achieved a significant reduction in blindness throughout the Commonwealth. Through its support of manpower and infrastructure development, it is laying the foundations of national eye care programmes which reach out to those who would otherwise have no access to such facilities. In this respect, it is making a significant contribution to the WHO's target of 'Health for All by the Year 2000'. For the first eight years of IAPB's work, the Society had the privilege of providing the Agency's central administration. The Society is currently providing the chairmanship and secretariat for the newly formed Consultative Group of non-governmental organizations to the WHO Programme for Prevention of Blindness.

Further information from: Royal Commonwealth Society for the Blind, Commonwealth House, Haywards Heath, West Sussex RH16 3AZ, UK.

Seva Foundation

Seva Foundation is an international service organization dedicated to relieving suffering, primarily through public health field programmes. Seva's major activities include support of prevention of blindness activities in Nepal and India. Seva was founded in 1978 by individuals who worked directly in, or were inspired by, the global eradication of smallpox, the first successful attempt in history to eliminate a disease world-wide. In 1982, Seva Service Society was founded as a vehicle for Seva's work in Canada.

At the invitation of His Majesty's Government of Nepal, Seva helped initiate the Nepal Blindness Programme in 1979. The goal of this nation-wide programme is to reduce preventable and curable blindness and to build Nepal's eye care infrastructure. The Programme is an international effort co-ordinated by His Majesty's Government and the World Health Organization.

Seva supports the national blindness programme in Nepal by: providing volunteer ophthalmologists and donated ophthalmic supplies and equipment, developing a national multimedia eye health education programme, and training ophthalmic personnel. Plans are underway to stimulate local production of eyeglasses. In conjunction with Nepal Netra Jyoti Sangh, Seva helped launch the Eye Care Subsidy Plan to encourage an increase in the number of sight-restoring procedures being provided.

In Nepal's Lumbini Zone, birthplace of Buddha, a model eye programme is being carried out with Seva support. Started in 1984, the programme has grown dramatically with the signing of bilateral agreements between Seva and the Government of Nepal.

The Nepal Blindness Survey showed that of Lumbini's 1.7 million people, roughly 40 000 are blind in one or both eyes. Approximately 133 000 (7.5 per cent) have potentially blinding trachoma and 48 000 have cataract. At least 700 children were found to suffer from eye problems due to insufficient vitamin A.

Zonal activities include satellite clinics, screening and surgical eye camps, and the establishment of a 35-bed hospital. Three full-time ophthalmologists carry out surgery and oversight. Ophthalmic assistants and hundreds of village volunteers help deliver eye care to the most remote areas of the zone.

In India, Seva supports the remarkable efforts of the Aravind Eye Hospital in Madurai. During its first 10 years, Aravind has provided over 1 million out-patient visits and performed more than 100 000 eye operations. Seva provides supplies and equipment, consultants in a variety of medical and public health disciplines, grants to cover food and transportation costs for cataract patients, and funds to support development of new satellite hospitals and clinics. Dr G. Venkataswamy, Director of Aravind Eye Hospital is a Seva Foundation Board member.

In addition to prevention of blindness efforts, Seva supports reforestation projects in Costa Rica, Lesotho, and the United States, public health activities among Native Americans in South Dakota and efforts to enhance economic independence among

Guatemalan refugees in Mexico. Seva also acts as a catalyst for the expression of service in North America by conducting regional conferences and developing local groups which provide compassionate action within their own communities.

Seva receives funds from individual donations, foundation grants, corporations, and a variety of fund-raising efforts including lecture series and concerts.

Further information from: Seva Foundation, 108 Spring Lake Drive, Chelsea, Michigan 48118, USA.

World Blind Union

The World Blind Union (WBU) is an international non-governmental organization composed of representatives of national associations of the blind and agencies serving the blind. It has come into being as an efficient organization after the historic decision taken in Riyadh, Saudi Arabia on 26 October 1984, when the long-cherished dream of many blind people was realized by the dissolution of both the International Federation of the Blind (IFB) and the World Council for the Welfare of the Blind (WCWB), and the establishment of the WBU. It was registered on 20 December 1984 with the authorities in Paris in accordance with the French Law of 1 July 1901. The headquarters of the Union are located in Paris, France.

The purposes of the Union are: to work for the prevention of blindness and the advancement of the well-being of blind and visually impaired people, with the goal of equalization of opportunities and full participation in society by special, legal, or administrative measures; to strengthen the self-awareness of blind persons; to develop their personalities, self-respect, and sense of responsibility; and to provide an international form for the exchange of knowledge and experience in the field of blindness.

The members of the World Blind Union are grouped into seven geographical Unions, which serve as bridges between the National Members and the Union of the World level, and further the work of the Union at the regional level. The geographical regions are: Africa, Asia, Europe, the Middle East, North America, Latin America, and East Asia Pacific.

The functions of WBU cover a wide range of interests in society. In its efforts to fulfil these functions, the Executive Committee of the Union has created several standing committees. These committees consist of experts in the field and represent a global view on the issues of blind.

The Standing Committees maintains regular contacts with the United Nations, specialized agencies, and other international non-governmental organizations.

The General Assembly of WBU meets every four years to determine general policies, elects the Executive Committee and the officers, considers their recommendations, approve reports of activities, and adopts the budget of the Union.

The Bulletin of the World Blind Union, *The World Blind*, is published quarterly in English in print and Braille and is recorded on cassette. Translations into French and Spanish are also available.

The World Blind Union has since its foundation asserted that the cause, control, and prevention of blindness have always been of great concern and constitute one of the major objectives of this world body. Through its concerned committee and members throughout the world, in co-operation and co-ordination with the World Health Organization (WHO), the International Agency for the Prevention of Blindness (IAPB), and the national organizations working in this field, it has taken necessary, effective, and concrete measures for protection of sight and prevention against blinding diseases all over the world.

The WBU, in conjunction with the Regional Bureau of the Middle East Committee for the Affairs of the Blind and in co-operation with the Saudi Ophthalmological Society, is planning to implement a comprehensive and integrated programme for eradicating trachoma, an important cause of blindness in the Kingdom of Saudi Arabia. This programme will be carried out over a period of five years, according to a phased plan and timetable for control and eradication of trachoma in the Kingdom.

Further information from: World Blind Union, PO Box 3465, Riyadh, Saudi Arabia.

Appendix A

WHO REGIONAL OFFICES, COLLABORATING CENTRES
FOR THE PREVENTION ON BLINDNESS, AND MEMBER
NATIONS BY REGION

WHO Regional Offices

World Health Organization
Regional Office for Africa
PO Box 6
Brazzaville
Congo

Pan American Health Organization
Regional Office of the
World Health Organization
525 23rd Street, NW
Washington, DC, 20037
USA

World Health Organization
Regional Office for the
Eastern Mediterranean
PO Box 1517
Alexandria 21511
Egypt

World Health Organization
Regional Office for Europe
8 Scherfigsvej
DK-2100 Copenhagen
Denmark

World Health Organization
Regional Office for
South-East Asia
World Health House
New Delhi 1.10.002
India

World Health Organization
Regional Office for the
Western Pacific
United Nations Avenue
PO Box 2932
Manila 2801
Philippines

WHO Collaborating Centres for the Prevention of Blindness

AFRICAN REGION

Institut d'Ophtalmologie
tropicale de l'Afrique
BP 248
Bamako
Mali
(Directeur: Dr P. Vingtain)

REGION OF THE AMERICAS

International Center for
Epidemiologic
and Preventive Ophthalmology
The Dana Center
Wilmer Institute
600 North Wolfe Street
Baltimore
Maryland 21205
USA
(Director: Professor Alfred
Sommer)

National Eye Institute
National Institutes of Health
Bldg. 31, Rm. 6A03
Bethesda
Maryland 20892
USA
(Director: Dr Carl Kupfer)

Dr Rodolfo Robles V Eye and Ear
    Hospital
National Committee for the Blind
    and Deaf
4a Avenida 2–28, Zona 1
Guatemala City
Guatemala
(Director: Dr F. Beltranena)

Centro Oftalmologico 'Luciano
    E. Barrere'
Hospital Santo Toribio de
    Mogrovejo
Ancash 1271
Lima
Peru
(Director: Dr F. Contreras)

Francis I. Proctor Foundation
    for Research in Ophthalmology
University of California
    San Francisco
San Francisco
California 94143
USA
(Director: Dr C. R. Dawson)

Serviço de Oftalmologica Sanitária
Secretaria de Estado da Saude
Av. Dr Enéas de Carvalho Aguiar
    No. 188
8° Andar
Caixa Postal 8027
São Paulo, SP 05403
Brazil
(Director: Dr O. Monteiro de
    Barros)

EASTERN MEDITERRANEAN
REGION

Institut d'Ophtalmologie
Bab-Saadoun
Tunis
Tunisia
(Directeur: Professeur M. T.
    Daghfous)

King Khaled Eye Specialist
    Hospital
PO Box 7191
Riyadh 11462
Saudi Arabia
(Director: Dr Ihsan Badr)

EUROPEAN REGION

International Centre for Eye
    Health
Department of Preventive
Ophthalmology
Institute of Ophthalmology
University of London
27/29 Cayton Street
London EC1V 9EJ
UK
(Director: Professor Barrie
    R. Jones)

Department of Viral and Allergic
    Eye Diseases
Helmholtz Research Institute of
    Ophthalmology
Sadovaja-Chernogriazslakaj 14/19
Moscow 103064
USSR
(Director: Professor I. F.
    Maitchouk)

SOUTH-EAST ASIA REGION

Dr Rajendra Prasad Centre
  for Ophthalmic Sciences
All-India Institute of Medical
  Sciences
Ansari Nagar
New Delhi 110016
India
(Director: Professor Madan Mohan)

WESTERN PACIFIC REGION

Department of Ophthalmology
Juntendo University School of
Medicine
3–1–3 Hongo
Bunkyo-ku
Tokyo 113
Japan
(Director: Professor
  A. Nakajima)

WHO Member Nations by Region

Countries with national prevention of blindness committees affiliated with
the IAPB are in bold type.

The 135 countries to which the *IAPB News* is mailed are indicated by
asterisks.

AFRICAN REGION

Algeria*, Angola, Benin*, **Botswana***, Burkina Faso*, Burundi,
Cameroon*, Cape Verde, Central African Republic, Chad, Comoros,
Congo*, Equatorial Guinea, Ethiopa*, Gabon, Gambia*, **Ghana***,
Guinea*, Guinea-Bissau, Ivory Coast*, **Kenya***, Lesotho*,
Liberia*, Madagascar*, **Malawi***, **Mali***, Mauritania*, Mauritius*,
Mozambique*, Niger, **Nigeria***, Rwanda*, São Tome and Principe,
Senegal*, Seychelles, Sierra Leone, **South Africa***, Swaziland*,
United Republic of Tanzania*, Togo, **Uganda***, Zaire, **Zambia***,
Zimbabwe*.

(The *IAPB News* is also mailed to the Canary Islands.)

REGION OF THE AMERICAS

Antigua and Barbuda*, **Argentina***, Bahamas, **Barbados***, Belize*,
Bolivia*, **Brazil***, **Canada***, Chile*, **Colombia***, **Costa Rica***, Cuba*,
Dominica*, Dominican Republic*, Ecuador*, El Salvador*, Grenada,
Guatemala*, Guyana*, **Haiti***, Honduras*, Jamaica*, Mexico*,
Nicaragua, Panama*, Paraguay*, **Peru***, St. Christopher and Nevis*,
St. Lucia, St. Vincent and The Grenadines*, Surinam, Trinidad and
Tobago*, **United States of America***, Uruguay*, **Venezuela***.

(The *IAPB News* is also mailed to Anguilla, Montserrat, Netherlands
Antilles, Puerto Rico, and Turks and Caicos Islands.)

EASTERN MEDITERRANEAN REGION

Afghanistan*, Bahrain*, Cyprus*, Democratic Yemen, Djibouti*,
Egypt*, Iran*, Iraq*, Jordan*, Kuwait*, Lebanon*, Libyan Arab

Jawahiriya*, **Morocco***, Oman, **Pakistan***, Qatar, **Saudi Arabia***, **Somalia***, **Sudan***, Syrian Arab Republic*, **Tunisia***, United Arab Emirates*, Yemen Arab Republic*.

EUROPEAN REGION

Albania, Austria*, **Belgium***, Bulgaria*, Byelorussian SSR, Czechoslovakia*, **Denmark***, **Federal Republic of Germany***, **Finland***, **France***, **German Democratic Republic***, Greece*, Hungary*, Iceland, Ireland*, **Israel***, **Italy***, Luxembourg*, Malta*, Monaco, **The Netherlands***, **Norway***, **Poland***, Portugal*, Romania*, San Marino, **Spain***, **Sweden***, Switzerland*, Turkey*, Ukranian SSR, **Union of Soviet Socialist Republics***, **United Kingdom***, **Yugoslavia***.

(The *IAPB News* is also mailed to Gibraltar.)

SOUTH-EAST ASIA REGION

Bangladesh*, Bhutan, Burma*, Democratic People's Republic of Korea, **India***, **Indonesia***, Maldives, Mongolia, **Nepal***, **Sri Lanka***, Thailand*.

WESTERN PACIFIC REGION

Australia*, Brunei Darussalem*, **China***, Cook Islands, Democratic Kampuchea, **Fiji***, **Japan***, Kiribati, Lao People's Democratic Republic*, **Malaysia***, **New Zealand***, **Papua New Guinea***, Philippines*, **Republic of Korea***, Samoa, **Singapore***, Soloman Islands, Tonga, Vanuatu, Vietnam*.

(The *IAPB News* is also mailed to Hong Kong.)

Appendix B

IAPB OFFICERS, REGIONAL CO-CHAIRMEN, AND
EXECUTIVE BOARD MEMBERS, 1986–90

IAPB Officers

President:	Dr Carl Kupfer
Honorary President:	Sir John Wilson
Vice Presidents:	
Senior Vice President:	Prof. Akira Nakajima
Vice President:	Dr A. Edward Maumenee (President, International Federation of Ophthalmological Societies)
Vice President:	Sheikh Abdullah Al-Ghanim (President, World Blind Union)
Vice President:	Mr Alan Johns (Chairman, NGO Coordinating Committee)
Vice President:	Dr Arthur Lim
Treasurer:	Mr Jack W. Swartwood
Registrar/Secretary:	Dr Viggo Clemmesen

Regional Co-chairmen

AFRICAN REGION

Chairman:	Dr M. C. Chirambo
Co-chairman for East:	Mr S. K. Tororei
Co-chairman for West:	[to be announced]

REGION OF THE AMERICAS

Co-chairman for North:	Mrs Virginia Boyce
Co-chairman for North:	Mr John M. Palmer III
Chairman for South:	Dr Francisco C. Contreras
Co-chairman for South:	Dr Fernando Beltranena
Co-chairman for South:	Dr Newton Kara-Jose
Co-chairman for South:	Dr Eugenio Maul

EASTERN MEDITERRANEAN REGION

Chairman: Sheikh Abdullah Al-Ghanim

EUROPEAN REGION

Co-chairman for East: Prof. Eduard S. Avetisov
Co-chairman for West: Prof. Asbjorn Tonjum

SOUTH-EAST ASIA REGION

Chairman: Dr. R. Pararajasegaram
Co-chairman: Dr Rajendra Vyas
Co-chairman: Dr S. R. K. Malik

WESTERN PACIFIC REGION

Co-chairman: Dr Arthur Lim
Co-chairman: Prof. Frank A. Billson
Co-chairman: Prof. Akira Nakajima

Executive Board Members

Group A: Appointed by the International Council of Ophthalmology, the executive body of the International Federation of Ophthalmic Societies.

Member	*Alternate*
Dr A. Edward Maumanee	Prof. Winifred Mao
Dr Carl Kupfer	Dr William S. Hunter
Prof. Akira Nakajima	Prof. Madan Mohan
Prof. Frank Billson	Dr C. O. Quarcoopome
Dr Arthur Lim	Dr Siva Reddy

Group B: Appointed by the President of the World Blind Union (WBU), subject to confirmation by the WBU Executive Board. The WBU was formed by the International Federation of the Blind (IFB) and the World Council for the Welfare of the Blind (WCWB) in 1984.

Member	*Alternate*
Sheikh Abdullah Al-Ghanim	Shahid Ahmed Memon
Dr Franz Sonntag	Mr Horst Stolper
Sra. Dorina de Gouvea Nowill	Sra. E. Molina de Stahl
Dr Rajendra Vyas	Mr Suresh C. Ahuja
Mr William Gallagher	Mr David Blyth

Group C: National Members

Member	*Alternate*
Prof. Adenike Abiose (Nigeria)	Prof. Ridha Mabrouk (Tunisia)

Prof. Eduard S. Avetisov
(USSR)   [to be announced]
Mr William Brohier (Malaysia)   Dr Bon Sool Koo
                                         (South Korea)

Prof. Cheng Hu (China)   [to be announced]
Dr M. C. Chirambo (Malawi)   Mr S. K. Tororei (Kenya)
Dr Viggo Clemmesen   Dr J. P. Herbecq
(Denmark)   (Belgium)
Dr Francisco Contreras (Peru)   Mr Wilbur Williams
                                         (Jamaica)
Prof. Newton Kara José   Dr Fernando Beltranena
(Brazil)   (Guatemala)
Dr S. R. K. Malik (India)   Prof. Rabiul Husain
                                         (Bangladesh)
Mr John M. Palmer III (USA)   Mrs Virginia Boyce
                                         (USA)
Dr Ram Prasad Pokhrel (Nepal)   Dr Wirasinghe (Sri
                                         Lanka)
Prof. Hadi El-Sheikh (Sudan)   Dr J. H. Wania (Pakistan)

Group D: Scientific disiplines other than ophthalmology.
Member   *Alternate*
Dr Alfred Sommer   Dr Fred Hollows
Dr Narong Sadudi   ⁻Dr Kazuichi Konyama
Dr Chandler Dawson   [to be announced]

Group E: A representative from each of the following international non-
governmental organizations.
Asian Foundation for the Prevention of Blindness (Mr Alan
Johns, acting)
Christoffel-Blindenmission (Mr P. G. Weiland)
Foresight (Maj.-Gen. Paul A. Cullen)
Helen Keller International (Mr John M. Palmer III)
International Eye Foundation (Mr Douglass Arbuckle)
International Organization Against Trachoma (Dr Gabriel
Coscas)
Operation Eyesight Universal (Mr A. T. Jenkyns)
Organization pour la Prevention de la Cécité (Dr A. Dubois-
Paulsen)
Royal Commonwealth Society for the Blind (Mr Alan Johns)
Seva Foundation (Dr Girija Brilliant)

Group F: Individual members by reason of an outstanding contribution
to international prevention of blindness activities:
Prof. Barrie R. Jones
Dr Bjorn Thylefors
Dr R. Pararajasegaram
Prof. G. Venkataswamy

Appendix C

CONSTITUTION OF THE INTERNATIONAL AGENCY FOR
THE PREVENTION OF BLINDNESS

ARTICLE I: Formation and name

1. *Formation*

An international, non-governmental organization is hereby created by
organizations concerned internationally with blindness and with ophthalmology to take over and expand the activities of the International Association for the Prevention of Blindness.

2. Name

The official name of the Agency shall be 'International Agency for the
Prevention of Blindness' (henceforward in this Constitution referred to as
'the Agency'). For non-official purposes, the Agency may use the name
'Vision International' or such other name as may be approved by the
General Assembly.

ARTICLE II: Commencement

The Agency comes into operation on the first day of January 1975, from
which date the International Association for the Prevention of Blindness
ceases to exist and all the assets and liabilities of the said Association are
transferred to the Agency.

ARTICLE III: Headquarters

The Headquarters of the Agency shall be located at a place designated by
the Executive Board.

ARTICLE IV: Purpose and powers

1. Purpose

The purpose of the Agency is to promote the prevention and cure of blindness (which expression unless the context otherwise indicates, shall include impaired vision) and to preserve sight.

2. Powers

The Agency may take any action which is conducive to the attainment of its purpose, including:

(a) To investigate and make known the causes, extent and consequences of blindness and to promote, support and encourage all or any measures designed to prevent, cure, reduce or remedy diseases, conditions and causes which produce blindness.

(b) To co-operate with the United Nations and its specialized agencies, with Governments and with national and international organizations concerned in any way with blindness and its prevention and to provide opportunities and facilities for such co-operation and for the co-ordination and development of the activities of co-operating organizations. To promote and support the establishment, maintenance and development of national and regional organizations and committees for the prevention and cure of blindness.

(c) To advance the science, practice and study of ophthalmology, to encourage research, and to foster international and multidisciplinary co-operation between scientists of different disciplines.

(d) To mobilize and assist in the mobilization of resources including the raising of funds, the acceptance of grants, bequests and gifts of all kinds, and the stimulation of governmental support for national and international action to prevent and cure blindness. To undertake and execute any trusts which may lawfully be undertaken by the Agency and to invest the funds of the Agency in such investments, securities and property as may be approved by the Executive Board.

(e) To promote the incorporation, registration and recognition of the Agency in any country of the world and to promote the establishment, maintenance and development of any trust, fund or organization whose objects are conducive or incidental to the attainment of the purpose of the Agency, provided that in any country in which the Agency is registered as a charity, the Agency shall not undertake any activity which is contrary to such charitable status.

(f) To collaborate with and support the activities of the World Council for the Welfare of the Blind, the International Federation of Ophthalmological Societies and to continue the activities of the International Association for the Prevention of Blindness.

(g) To engage and remunerate employees, to institute pension schemes and other appropriate benefits for employees, ex-employees and their dependents and to pay appropriate remuneration to any person whose services are required in connection with the activities of the Agency provided that no officer or member of the Executive Board shall receive any salary or remuneration other than reimbursement of expenses which, in the opinion of the Executive Board, are necessarily incurred in connection with the work of the Agency. The income and property of the Agency shall be applied solely towards the promotion of the purpose of the Agency and no portion thereof shall be paid or transferred by way of dividend, share, bonus or otherwise by way of profit to the members of the Agency apart from the payment in good faith of reasonable and proper remuneration to any member of the Agency in return for services actually rendered.

(h) To do all such other things as are incidental or conducive to the attainment of the Purpose of the Agency.

ARTICLE V: Members

1. Categories of membership

The Agency may have an unlimited number of members in the following categories:

(a) National Delegates, that is persons nominated for appointment as national delegates in accordance with the procedure prescribed in Article VI (1) of this Constitution.

(b) International Delegates, that is persons nominated for appointment as international delegates in accordance with the procedure prescribed in Article VI (3) of this Constitution.

(c) Representative Members, that is persons nominated for appointment as their representatives by organizations which do not have the right to nominate national or international delegates but to which the Executive Board or the General Assembly has accorded the right to nominate representative members.

(d) Ophthalmologists and Professional Members, that is individuals qualified as ophthalmologists or in some science or profession recognized by the Executive Board as appropriate for the purpose of according the status of professional membership.

(e) Associate Members, that is individuals to whom the Executive Board has accorded the status of associate membership.

(f) Honorary Members, that is individuals not exceeding fifty in number to whom the General Assembly has accorded the status of honorary membership either for life or for a stipulated period of years.

2. Financial contributions

The General Assembly shall delegate to the Executive Board authority to determine the financial contributions appropriate to each category of membership.

ARTICLE VI: Delegates

1. National delegates

National Delegates may be appointed from any country in which there exists a national committee or national organization (or any approved grouping of such committees and organizations) recognized by the Executive Board as entitled to appoint that country's national delegates. The Executive Board may withhold such recognition if it considers that the nominating committee, organization or group is insufficiently representative of the organizations and interests concerned with the prevention of blindness in that country.

2. Number of national delegates

The number of national delegates which may be nominated for appointment from any country shall be related to the size of that country's population as revealed in the most recent national census. A country with a population not exceeding five million may appoint one delegate. A country with a population of more than five million but not exceeding 20 million may appoint two delegates. A country with a population of more than 20 million but not exceeding 50 million may appoint four delegates. A country with a population of more than 50 million may appoint six delegates.

3. International delegates

The Executive Board may authorize an international non-governmental organization to nominate a representative for appointment as an international delegate. Before according such right of nomination, the Executive Board shall be satisfied that the organization concerned is international in scope and that it promotes, operates or co-ordinates a substantial programme for the prevention or cure of blindness.

ARTICLE VII: Commencement and termination of membership

1. Commencement

The Executive Board shall appoint a suitable person to act as Registrar and such Registrar shall maintain the register of all members of the Agency. All applications for membership shall be made in writing to the Registrar who, if satisfied that the applicant is qualified for membership in accordance with the provisions of Article V of this Constitution and that any appropriate financial contributions have been paid, shall enter the applicant's name in the register of members and the applicant shall thereupon assume the rights appropriate to the category of membership. Any person or organization whose application is refused by the Registrar or whose application is not proceeded with within three months, may appeal to the Executive Board or to a Committee of the Board authorized to consider such appeals and the decision of the Board or of such Committee shall be final.

2. Termination

A member's name shall be withdrawn from the register and membership shall cease if:
(a) Membership is terminated by the organization or committee which nominated the member a delegate or representative member.
(b) Any fianncial contribution appropriate to the category of membership shall remain unpaid for a period of twelve months.
(c) Membership is terminated by a resolution of the Executive Board in which event any financial contributions which have been paid in respect of the membership during the preceding year shall be refunded.

3. The Register

The Register of Members, or a true copy thereof, shall be kept at the Headquarters and shall be open to inspection during normal office hours by any member of the Agency.

ARTICLE VIII: The General Assembly

1. The first General Assembly shall be convened by the President not later than three years from the date on which the Agency comes into operation. Subsequent Assemblies shall be held at intervals not exceeding four years and at a time and place determined by the General Assembly or the Executive Board. The President, by giving two months' written notice to all members, may convene an Extraordinary General Assembly and shall convene such an Assembly if he is requested to do so by a majority of the members of the Executive Board or by a majority of the national and international delegates. General Assemblies shall, so far as possible, be held at a time and place likely to be convenient to a majority of the members having regard to the timing of other international conferences of ophthalmologists or of blind welfare workers.

2. Function

The General Assembly shall be the governing body of the Agency and its decisions shall determine the general policies by which the Agency shall seek to achieve its purpose. The General Assembly shall elect the officers and the Executive Board in accordance with the procedure prescribed in Article X and XI of this Constitution. It shall review the work of the Executive Board, approve the general report, accounts and budget of the Agency, and shall regulate the Agency's relationship with other organizations.

3. Resolutions

The General Assembly shall have the power to adopt special and general resolutions. A special resolution of the General Assembly is a resolution which concerns:
(a) the amendment of the Constitution;

(b) the number of members in each group of the Executive Board as prescribed in Article XI of this Constitution and the election or appointment of members in Groups A, B and C of the Executive Board;

(c) approval of the financial estimates of the Agency;

(d) the dissolution of the Agency.

A general resolution is a resolution which is concerned with any other business of the General Assembly. In the event of disagreement whether a resolution is special or general, the decision of the President or, in his absence, of the officer presiding as Chairman of the Assembly, shall be final. Except with the approval of the Executive Board, no special resolution shall be proposed in the General Assembly unless it has previously been submitted in writing to the Secretary-General at least eight weeks before the commencement of the General Assembly.

ARTICLE IX: Votes in the General Assembly

1. Votes on general resolutions

Every registered member of the Agency may attend and participate in the business of the General Assembly and may exercise one vote on any general resolution.

2. Votes on special resolutions

Only national delegates, international delegates and members of the Executive Board may vote on a special resolution as defined in Article VIII (3) of this Constitution.

3. Limitation

On any resolution not more than fifteen per cent of the votes shall be cast by members who are citizens of the same country. If in any General Assembly more than fifteen per cent of the members with voting rights are citizens of the same country, these members shall decide between themselves on the limitation of their voting rights in accordance with this Clause and should they fail to agree, the matter shall be decided by lot.

4. Quorum

At any General Assembly, forty members shall constitute a quorum for the purpose of considering a general resolution and thirty members with voting rights on a special resolution shall constitute a quorum for the purpose of considering a special resolution.

5. All resolutions at a General Assembly shall be decided by a majority of the votes cast except for resolutions to amend the Constitution or dissolve the Agency, which shall be decided in accordance with the procedure prescribed in Article XIII and Article XIV of this Constitution. Voting may be viva voce, by show of hands or by ballot which may be secret if so decided by the President or, in his absence, by the officer presiding as

Chairman of the Assembly. Unless otherwise decided by the General Assembly, the election of an officer of the Agency shall be by secret ballot. Between meetings of the General Assembly questions which, in the view of the Executive Board lie outside the powers committed to that Board, may be decided by postal ballot of all members qualified to vote on the question at issue.

6. Proxies

A national delegate who is unable to attend a session of the General Assembly may authorize another member of his national delegation to exercise a proxy vote on his behalf. Written notice of such proxy must be given to the Secretary-General before the commencement of the session of the General Assembly at which such proxy vote will be exercised. No delegate shall exercise more than two proxy votes.

7. In the event of an equality of votes on any resolution the President or, in his absence, the officer presiding as Chairman of the Assembly, may exercise a second or casting vote.

ARTICLE X: Officers

1. The Officers of the Agency shall be: President, one or more Vice-Presidents, Treasurer, Secretary-General and such other officers as may from time to time be appointed by special resolution of the General Assembly. If more than one Vice-President is appointed, one of them shall be designated as the Senior Vice-President.

2. Officers shall be elected by general resolution of the General Assembly from amongst the members elected or appointed at that Assembly as members of the Executive Board. Unless otherwise determined by the General Assembly, the President and Senior Vice-President shall be elected from among the membership of Groups A and B of the Executive Board, one such officer from each Group. The officers of the Agency shall hold office until the conclusion of the next General Assembly when they shall retire from office but, subject to the provisions of Clause 3 of this Article with regard to the period of office of the President, shall be eligible for re-election.

3. The President, in co-operation with the Officers, shall give leadership in the activities of the Agency and in the formulation of its policy. The President shall have the right to preside at all meetings of the General Assembly and of the Executive Board. No person shall hold the office of President for a consecutive period exceeding eight years but, should this period elapse between meetings of the General Assembly, the President may continue in office on a temporary basis until the conclusion of the next General Assembly at which the new President shall be elected.

4. The Vice-President, or should thereby more than one Vice-President, the Senior Vice-President, shall act as assistant to the President and, in the President's absence, shall preside at meetings of the General Assembly and of the Executive Board. In the event of the incapacity, resignation or death of the President, the Senior Vice-President shall assume the duties of the President pending the appointment of a new President by the General Assembly. If the President for the time being is not a qualified ophthalmologist, the Senior Vice-President or other qualified officer designated by the Executive Board, shall act as the Agency's representative on the International Council of Ophthalmology.

5. The Treasurer and Secreatary-General shall undertake the duties appropriate to their respective offices and such additional duties as may be specified by the Executive Board or the President. In the event of disagreement about the duties of the respective Officers, the decision of the President shall be final.

6. The Officers collectively shall act, under the chairmanship of the President, as an Executive Committee of the Executive Board with power, between meetings of the Board, to make decisions necessary for the continuation and advancement of the work of the Agency and to undertake such additional duties as may be assigned to them by the Executive Board.

ARTICLE XI: Executive Board

1. Each General Assembly shall elect an Executive Board whose members shall serve until the conclusion of the next General Assembly when they shall retire from office but be eligible for re-election.

2. The Executive Board shall consist of the following groups of members:

Group A. Members appointed by special resolution on the nomination of the International Council of Ophthalmology to represent organizations concerned with ophthalmology and with the prevention of blindness.

Group B. Members appointed by special resolution on the nomination of the World Council for the Welfare of the Blind to represent organizations for and of the blind.

Group C. Members elected by special resolution to represent the national delegates appointed in accordance with the provisions of Article VI of this Constitution.

Group D. Members elected by general resolution to represent scientific disciplines other than ophthalmology.

Group E. Members elected by general resolution to represent international non-governmental organizations whose activities contribute to the attainment of the purpose of the Agency.

Group F. Members elected by general resolution in recognition of the individual contribution which they can make to the work of the Agency.

3. Until otherwise determined by special resolution of the General Assembly, the maximum number of members in each of the Groups prescribed in Clause 2 of this Article, shall be:

Group A Five	Group D Four
Group B Five	Group E Four
Group C Five	Group F Four

4. Alternates

For each member of the Executive Board, an alternate may be appointed who, on behalf of and at the request of the member, may attend and vote at any meeting of the Board from which the member is absent. Each alternate shall be appointed by the same procedure as that described in Clause 2 of this Article for the appointment or election of the member whose alternate he is. No alternate shall perform any of the duties of an Officer.

5. Vacancies

Between General Assemblies, any member of the Executive Board who vacates office shall be succeeded by the alternate and the Executive Board shall thereupon appoint another suitable person to service as alternate. In the event of the incapacity, resignation or death of an Officer other than the President, the Executive Board may appoint one of its members to perform the duties of the vacant office until the next meeting of the General Assembly.

ARTICLE XII: Powers of the Executive Board

1. The Executive Board shall be responsible for interpreting the decisions and policies adopted by the General Assembly. It shall administer, manage and control the affairs, finances and property of the Agency and in so doing shall be authorized to take any action not specifically reserved for the General Assembly. It shall supervise the activity of the Officers and employees of the Agency and shall have the right at all times to receive reports on their activity.

2. The Executive Board shall decide on the time and place of its meetings which shall be held at least once every two years. At any meeting of the Board, a quorum shall consist of half the members for the time being of the Board or eight members, whichever number is least. An alternate attending a meeting on behalf of a member, shall count as a member for the purpose of the quorum.

3. The Executive Board may decide on any matter within its competence by:
(a) The agreement of a majority of the members present at a meeting at which there is a quorum as defined in Clause 2 of this Article.
(b) The agreement of a majority of the members voting in a postal ballot which has been circulated to all members at least six weeks before the

votes are counted and in which votes are recorded by not fewer than half the members of the Executive Board or by eight members, whichever is least.

In the event of an equality of votes, the President or officer presiding as Chairman of the Executive Board may have a second or casting vote.

4. Committees

The Executive Board may appoint Committees for any purpose with such terms of reference and duties as it may decide. Such Committees shall consist of members of the Agency but non-members may be co-opted in a consultative or advisory capacity.

5. Financial control

It shall be the duty of the Executive Board to ensure the maintenance of an efficient system of accountancy and financial control and at all times to cause expenditure to be regulated within the income and resources of the Agency. The accounts and balance sheet of the Agency shall be audited annually by a professionally qualified auditor and copies of the accounts and balance sheet together with a report on the activities of the Agency, shall be made available annually to all registered members of the Agency and to an authorities entitled to receive such accounts and reports.

6. Nominations

At the time of the General Assembly, the Executive Board shall be entitled to propose, for the consideration of the Assembly or of any nominations committee appointed by the Assembly, the names of persons it considers suitable for nomination as officers or as members of the Executive Board. These nominations shall in no way limit the freedom of choice of the Assembly.

ARTICLE XIII: Constitutional amendments

1. This Constitution may be amended:

(a) By a special resolution of the General Assembly (as defined in Article VIII (3) of this Constitution), adopted by a majority of not less than two thirds of the members present and voting on the resolution.

(b) With the consent of the Executive Board by a postal ballot of all members entitled to vote on a special resolution provided that not less than two thirds of the votes cast are in favour of the proposed amendment.

2. A Constitutional amendment may be proposed by the Executive Board or by not less than five members of the Agency. Any amendment proposed for consideration by the General Assembly shall be submitted in writing to the Secretary-General at least three months before the commencement of the General Assembly at which the amendment is to be considered.

ARTICLE XIV: Dissolution

The dissolution of the Agency shall require a special resolution of the General Assembly proposed by the Executive Board and adopted by a majority of not less than two-thirds of the members present and voting on the resolution. In the event of bankruptcy and subject to any laws applicable to the Agency, the personal liability of any member of the Agency shall be limited to a maximum of U.S.$10. On the dissolution of the Agency, any remaining assets shall be disposed of in accordance with the recognized legal procedure of the country in which such assets are owned.

Appendix D

PROPOSAL FOR CATARACT-FREE ZONES IN LATIN AMERICA *8 May 1986*

Contents

I. Background

Over the past two decades the Pan-American Association of Ophthalmology (PAAO) has primarily been concerned with upgrading the level of professional education throughout Latin America. This effort has been highly successful, and the result has been a very high level of ophthalmologic practice in Latin America, equivalent to the best anywhere in the world.

Now that this has been accomplished, it is appropriate for PAAO to undertake a broadened scope of activities. For example, there are increasing demands in Latin America—and for that matter throughout the world—for improved access for all people to better health care. Although new technology has in many cases made it more feasible in theory to respond to these demands, in actuality the high cost of such advances has frequently made such care all the more inaccessible to the poor.

In the United States the American Academy of Ophthalmology has launched the National Eye Care Project, which in its pilot phase was highly successful in reaching medically underserved elderly individuals. This project has recently been expanded to include the entire population. In Latin America, many governments believe that eye care should be a major part of general health care, but this has not yet been achieved on a wide scale.

To meet the challenge of providing high quality medical eye care to all who need it, there is need for new approaches—ones which represent a departure from traditional methods of health care delivery. One such approach, which could be engendered and co-ordinated by PAAO, is the concept of Cataract-Free Zones. This concept was first discussed and endorsed by PAAO's Executive Board at the Pan-American Congress of Ophthalmology, held 28 September–3 October 1985 in San Francisco, California. The Board agreed to hold a planning meeting for a pilot effort on 1–4 April 1986 at the National Institutes of Health to be jointly sponsored by PAAO and the United States' National Eye Institute (NEI) and Fogarty International Centre. The meeting was held as scheduled, and participants included PAAO and NEI officials and staff, prominent Latin American ophthalmologists, officials of the Pan-American Health Organization, staff of Helen Keller International, and experts in operations research and cataract intervention programmes. (See Attachment A of this Proposal for list of participants.)

This document contains the outcome of that meeting and proposes demonstration projects for defined areas within a limited population in two Latin American countries, Brazil and Peru. The goal is to reduce the level of cataract blindness within these areas to a minimum within a specified period of time. One fortunate aspect of such a project is that all the necessary technology is in place. But, as has been noted, technology alone will not achieve the goal. What must be worked out in some degree of detail is the best approach to bringing that technology to the population and vice versa. If such demonstration projects are successful, they can be expanded and replicated elsewhere in Latin America. The need is great, but the cost must be low. Our goal is to convey the idea that this type of effort, the details of which may vary within and among communities, regions, and countries, must be incorporated into general health care within these countries and all of Latin America if we are to make a major impact on preventable blindness by the end of this century.

II. Introduction

It is important to stress that the proposed Cataract-Free Zones are neither intended nor designed to replace or interfere with existing eye care; rather, they are conceived as being an addition to current eye care programmes in the community and carefully tailored to serve the needs of the community in which they are established. The Cataract-Free Zone project aims at serving a targeted urban population, not the well-to-do, not those with access to the health care provided through organized labour, and not those served by social security hospitals, but those currently with little or no access to eye care. Of necessity, this will be a 'vertical' health care project while in its time-limited demonstration phase, but if continued the concept must be incorporated into the overall health care system.

An essential component of the project is evaluation. One cannot judge its success merely on the basis of the number of cataract operations performed; one must compare the total number of people blind from cataract before and after the intervention. The goal of the project is to achieve a designated level of cataract blindness eradication within some limited period of time. Evaluation will tell us the extent to which this has been accomplished.

It is important to stress that the concept of a Cataract-Free Zone does not imply just a one-time intervention, but an ongoing programme, once the backlog of unoperated cases has been substantially reduced, to maintain the number of cataract blind at a designated minimal level. To clear the backlog will require a tremendous effort, but once done it will be much easier to keep up with the new cases. In Latin America there is enough manpower to handle the new cases; but the health care system is not yet in a position to deal effectively with the backlog. Operations research is a tool that can be used to devise innovative, efficient approaches to reducing the backlog.

We need first to identify the cause of the backlog of cataract cases. Surveys have shown that 40 per cent of the population of Latin America do not have access to any health care. Because little is known about the existing infrastructure for specialized care, it will be hard to know what course to follow after the demonstration project is completed. Thus, in parallel with the demonstration project, it will be important to investigate what is already going on in terms of health services to support cataract intervention. One important consideration is the attitude of Latin American ophthalmologists who, in general, are not oriented to community service. In order for such efforts as the Cataract-Free Zone to succeed, these attitudes will have to change. In this the PAAO can play an important role, particularly in influencing newly trained ophthalmologists. Governments too, in many instances, must change their attitudes and be supportive of non-traditional public health approaches.

Almost anywhere in the developing world, cataract is a bottleneck to prevention of blindness. Most hospitals will carry out a maximum of 15 to 20 cataract operations a day. Barriers to raising this capacity include a limit on beds and restrictive standards concerning the required length of post-operative hospitalization. One overarching limiting factor is that most developing nations have not yet adopted out-patient cataract surgery as the norm.

Knowledgeable Latin American ophthalmologists do not believe that the backlog of unoperated cases of cataract in their countries is due primarily to ignorance; it is likely that most people do know about the benefits of cataract surgery, but many have no means of accessing such care. Nonetheless, public education will be a necessary component of the Cataract-Free Zone project because many poor people have no doubt been discouraged in the past from seeking such care and will now have to be convinced that they should seek it.

Urban areas have been selected for the establishment of the demonstration Cataract-Free Zones. While the needs are undoubtedly great in rural areas as well, it is considered premature to approach rural areas as well, it is considered premature to approach rural areas at this time because a cataract care infrastructure, upon which these projects will depend, does not generally exist in such areas at present. Indeed, contemporary emphasis in public health in general is being placed increasingly on urban areas; rural migrants to the cities have become the most medically under-served populations in many countries.

The Peru site encompasses the entire city of Chimbote, with a population of around 240 000. The prevalence of cataract blindness in this population is estimated to be 1000 to 1200 cases. In Brazil, an impoverished, medically under-served portion of the city of Campinas will be selected. The zone will be defined to include 100 000 people, but if the cataract yield is below 500 cases, it will be expanded.

III. Project goal/objective

The goal of each Cataract-Free Zone project is to demonstrate a replicable means to ascertain and clear the cataract backlog (prevalence) in a Latin American urban area using the techniques of house-to-house visual acuity screening, out-patient surgery, and in-home community follow-up. Such an effort will include generating a sufficient level of community/government commitment and involvement to maintain continuity of cataract identification and treatment in the area. Stated in evaluable terms, the project objective is to reduce within one year in a defined urban district the backlog of cataract blindness—defined as 20/200 (or 6/60) best-corrected visual acuity or less—by a minimum of 70 per cent in those aged 50 and older by restoring corrected vision to 20/40 (or 6/12) or better.

The demonstration projects must be designed in a cost-effective manner if they are to represent replicable approaches to the cataract-blind problem. Each project must, at an acceptable level of cost, maximize effectiveness in (A) its *search* for all cataract-blind individuals, (B) its ability to obtain patient *consent* for examination and surgery, (C) its *logistics* whereby patients, medical personnel, and facilities are brought together, and (D) its surgical *intervention* to restore sight. Each of the four components has measurable goals associated with them which represent the minimum acceptable level to define success. However, in order to achieve the overall project goal of 70 per cent reduction in cataract blindness, some of the component minimum goals must be exceeded.

Of particular importance is the proposal to demonstrate the techniques of house-to-house visual acuity screening, out-patient surgery, and in-home/community follow-up. The house-to-house survey, which will follow a mass education campaign, is the search scheme that will be used to ensure that all cataract-blind individuals in the target population are identified. This initial person-to-person contact with all prospective patients is also important in increasing the percentage of cataract-blind that consent to the eye examination and, if indicated, surgery. By arranging transportation to the surgery site (hospital) and by conducting follow-up examinations in the home and at convenient community locations, the complexity and inconvenience of logistical factors will be reduced. The surgical intervention itself will be done on an out-patient basis to reduce cost while maintaining safety and effectiveness.

The following sections address the components of search, consent, logistics, and intervention. For each, the associated problem being faced is stated, the objective to be achieved is defined in evaluable terms, and a proposed approach is outlined. Each project will have its own unique features, which are noted in instances of particular importance. Generally, the differences unique to Campinas, Brazil are shown in parentheses. Where numerical values are shown, the Chimbote values precede the Campinas values which are in parentheses.

Local personnel must be involved in extending the planning to a detailed operational level appropriate to the locale (preparation of the Manual of Operations). The endorsement and approval of affected community groups, government organizations, and health provider organizations is also necessary.

IV. Search

A. *problem*
The search problem is to identify the cataract blind over age 50 within the area of the designated Cataract-Free Zone.

1. Target city: Chimbote, Peru (Campinas, Brazil).
2. Target population: entire city population of 240 602 (100 000 out of a city population of 900 000 people).
3. Population age 50 or over: 20 000 to 24 000 (13 000).
4. Expected cataract blind (20/200 or worse) over age 50: 1000 to 1200 cases (600 cases).

B. *Objective*
The search objective is to identify 95 per cent of the cataract blind within four months of the start of the project.

C. *approach*
The search for cataract blind will be conducted using a mass publicity campaign followed by a door-to-door household survey. The campaign by itself is not expected to be sufficiently effective in reaching 95 per cent of the cataract blind, thus the survey. The role of the campaign is to inform the general population about cataract blindness and the upcoming house-to-house survey and to encourage their co-operation. Through the survey, every household will be contacted on a person-to-person basis.

1. Mass publicity campaign

The campaign will consist of radio and television messages and community posters. It may be possible to obtain the financial support of industry for this. Preceding the campaign, it will be necessary to solicit the co-operation of the city government, volunteer organizations (such as Lions and Rotary Clubs), churches, and schools.

The message of the campaign will be directed toward:

(a) describing what a cataract is,
(b) pointing out that cataract is treatable and vision lost therefrom can be restored,
(c) informing the community that a house-to-house blindness survey will take place and minimizing distrust, and
(d) recruiting neighbourhood volunteers.

The campaign schedule will entail one month for preparation of materials and solicitation of community support and co-operation. The campaign itself will take place over a three- to four-week period prior to the start of the survey and then possibly continue at a reduced level of intensity during the survey period.

Although not proposed as part of this study, the effectiveness of the campaign could be evaluated (by an independent group) by randomly sampling those over the age of 50 to determine if they were aware of the campaign message. It is possible that the campaign publicity will attract cataract-blind people from outside the target area. In this event, the project will provide services to these individuals. The following resources are required for the campaign:

Project director, Dr F. Contreras (Dr N. Kara-Jose): 10% time.
Campaign/survey co-ordinator: 100% time.
Staff ophthalmologist: 10–20% time.
Development of presentation and campaign materials and audiovisuals.

2. House-to-house blindness survey

Based on an estimate of five occupants per house, the house-to-house survey is expected to cover 51 000 houses (20 000 houses). Each house will be visited by a survey team that is expected to:

(a) identify blind persons over age 50,
(b) convince the blind person to consent to an eye examination,
(c) follow-up to ensure that the examination was done, and
(d) provide referral suggestions for other ophthalmic problems.

Each survey team will consist of one paid member and one neighbourhood volunteer to function as an assistant. The volunteer will work with the paid team member only within the volunteer's neighbourhood. When the team moves to another neighbourhood, a new volunteer will be recruited. The paid member will take part in a two-day survey training session. The survey implementation period is scheduled to be of four-months duration and preceded by a two-month planning/preparation period which overlaps with the publicity campaign period.

Each survey team will work 40 to 50 hours per week. Assuming that on the average two houses per hour can be surveyed per team, each team will survey 400 houses per month. It will require 30 teams (15 teams) to complete the survey of all households within the scheduled four-month survey period. The project complement of survey teams will visit 500 houses (250 houses) per day with an expected cataract yield of 15(8) cases per day. Each team will identify an average of one cataract every other day.

For each household, a data collection form will be completed. Information to be collected will include:

(a) address of house,

(b) number of people over 50 who normally live there,

(c) name of cataract blind person,

(d) local resident or outsider (if blind person),

(e) age of blind person,

(f) sex of blind person, and

(g) visual acuity < 20/200 (yes or no).

Visual acuity will be checked by the survey team using a 'tumbling E' eye chart. A pinhole will be used to rule out refractive defects. Those determined to be possibly cataract blind will be requested to visit a clinic/ mobile exam unit for a more complete eye examination.

The following are the resource requirements for the survey:

- Campaign/survey coordinator: 100% time.
- Survey planning and preparation assistant: 2 months.
- Survey team members: 30 (15) for period of 5 months.
- 200 (100) volunteers.
- Materials: data forms, consent text, eye chart, flashlight, pinhole, logo T-shirts.

V. Decision/consent

A. problem

Potential project beneficiaries must make a conscious decision. They must consent first to the eye examination and then, if indicated, to cataract surgery. A variety of factors may deter the individual from consenting to the interventions: fear, religion (fate), geography, time, family support, and cost. Also, those with visual acuity near 20/200 may not perceive a need for surgery. The project is designed to overcome these barriers to consent thorough participant persuasion, logistical convenience, and full subsidy of costs. Potential beneficiaries must be convinced of the benefits of cataract surgery.

B. objective

The consent objectives are to obtain examination consent from 95 per cent of the survey positive cases within two weeks of the household visit and to obtain surgical consent from 80 per cent of the examination positives within four weeks of the examination.

C. *approach*

1. Eye examination consent

The household survey teams function as the primary exam consent team. Through the use of prepared consent materials, they will attempt to convince those with visual acuity equal to or less than 20/200 and no apparent refractive deficiencies to consent to an eye examination. Those not reporting for the examination within one week will be re-visited by the neighbourhood volunteer. If the volunteer's offer to accompany the individual to the exam station does not produce results within another week, a final visit by a consent team social worker will take place before further exam consent attempts are abandoned.

Social worker expertise is required for the consent function, including surgical consent efforts and other miscellaneous patient support:

2. Eye examination

The eye examinations will take place over a five-month period. The first four months will overlap the survey period with the fifth month extending beyond it.

(a) The exam protocol will consist of:
- visual acuity with pinhole,
- light projection with colour perception,
- external eye exam,
- intraocular pressure,
- slit lamp exam,
- compression of lacrimal sac, and
- for those for whom cataract surgery is indicated:
  1. blood pressure
  2. urinalysis
     (If either is positive, the patient will be referred for medical care.)

It is expected that 30 (12 to 15) exams will be conducted per day with 15 (8) cataracts diagnosed.

(b) The associated medical data collection will include:
- name,
- address,
- age,
- sex,
- identification number,
- date of examination,
- visual acuity,
- lens (cataract) opacity (for project evaluation),
- external examination findings,
- corneal condition,

-tonometry,
-retinal test results,
-lacrimal test results, and
-blood pressure and urinalysis results.

(c) The examination will require the following resources over a five month period:
-one ophthalmologist full time.
-one ophthalmic nurse full time.
-two aids full time.
-Materials: consumables, data collection, and office supplies.

3. Surgery consent

Obtaining surgery consent is the responsibility of the examination team with the assistance of the social worker. For examinees with cataract who consent, surgery will be scheduled within one week. Those who do not consent will be given three weeks to reconsider and consult with their families before the social worker visits to seek surgery consent.

The surgical consent period extends over the entire five-month examination period plus one additional month.

VI. Logistics

A. *problem*

A number of problemmatical logistical factors must be addressed if cataract surgery is to be provided to all potential beneficiaries in a cost-effective fashion. Cataract surgery and the events preceding and following it can impose an economic burden that is beyond the means of the potential beneficiary and entail a disruption of lifestyle that may be judged unacceptable by the beneficiary and/or his family. From the perspective of medical care providers, the accommodation of a significant number of additional cataract surgery cases within the existing infrastructure can also lead to disruption. A delivery system must be designed that is low in cost and yet effective in moving the patient through the intervention process.

B. *objective*

The logistics objective is to bring 98 per cent of those consenting to surgery to the hospital for cataract extraction within one week and provide all follow-up care in a home or community setting.

C. *approach*

1. Transport of patients to and from hospital

A bus and driver for the exclusive use of the project will be provided to transport patients to the hospital in the morning and return them to their homes at the end of the day after surgery. A volunteer will accompany the bus to provide assistance to patients, particularly to those without an accompanying family member. The bus and driver will also be available during the middle of the day to transport household survey positives to the eye examination station if required for obtaining consent.

Patient transportation will be required for a six-month period. The resource requirements are as follows:

(a) Vehicle for six months.

(b) Driver for six months.

(c) Fuel.

(d) Bus volunteers: 175 days, and logo T-shirts.

2. Post-surgery follow-up: Days 1 and 3

Follow-up of patients on post-surgery days 1 and 3 will be done in the home by a visiting nurse accompanied by a community volunteer. It is expected that the volunteer will provide a vehicle and be reimbursed for fuel costs. In-home care will minimize the logistical impact of surgery on the patient and family.

This in-home follow-up will take place during a six-month project time span. Resource requirements are as follows:

(a) Visiting nurse.

(b) Volunteers with nurse: 175 days, and logo T-shirts.

(c) Fuel for volunteer vehicles.

(d) Portable slit lamp.

(e) Medical supplies and materials: drops, steroids, and antibiotics

3. Post-surgery follow-up: Days 7 and 21

The follow-up routinely scheduled for days 7 and 21 need not occur precisely on those days. Indeed, it is planned that patients within the post-surgery interval of 7 to 13 days be grouped and examined on the same day of the week as will those 21 to 27 days post-surgery. This will simplify system logistics without sacrificing the quality of medical care.

The two different follow-up visits will take place in a community facility on a particular day of the week. The patients will not need to travel to the hospital and be merged into the myriad of activities competing for medical personnel and resources. Furthermore, by choosing a Saturday it should be possible to solicit volunteers to help with the once-a-week event. Glasses will be dispensed to those who are 7 to 13 days post-surgery and changed if necessary for those 21 to 27 days post-surgery. Aphakics will have an opportunity to visit and provide encouragement to one other.

It is planned that organization volunteers (such as Lions or Rotary Club members) with vehicles will be engaged to pick up all 7 to 13 and 21 to 27 day aphakics at their homes and return them after the follow-up examination. The volunteer organizations may also participate in the purchase and presentation of glasses, the latter perhaps could be done at a 'restoration of sight' ceremony. Based on 15 (8) patients receiving surgery per day, there will be approximately 150 (80) aphakics at each weekly event. From beginning to end, the follow-up period will span nearly seven months: the six-month surgery period plus an additional one month of follow-up at the end. The follow-up load will be less than that 150 (80) per week at the beginning and end of the period.

Resources needed for these weekly follow-up events are primarily examination personnel:

(a) One ophthalmologist.

(b) Three (two) ophthalmic nurses.

(c) One aid.

(d) Medical supplies and materials.

(e) Glasses with case.

4. Patient flow

The decision diagram (Attachment B) displays in logical sequence the series of decisions and intervention steps that the patient experiences as he or she 'flows' through the delivery system. The outcome for all identified blind people will be tracked by recording their progression through the sequence of survey exam consent → examination → surgery consent → surgical intervention. This data will provide the basis for evaluation of project effectiveness. The proposed data elements are:

(a) name/identification,

(b) address,

(c) age,

(d) sex,

(e) date of survey/house visit,

(f) date of exam consent,

(g) date of examination,

(h) date of surgical consent,

(i) surgical consent mode (examination, delayed, social worker), and

(j) date of surgery

VII. Intervention

A. problem
The surgical intervention problem is the cataract that requires safe removal.

B. objective
The objective of the surgical intervention procedure is to achieve at least a 95 per cent operative success rate using existing surgical resources. Success is defined as providing the aphakic with 20/40 or better vision.

C. approach

Chimbote   **Campinas**

Out-patient surgery (with some exceptions: one-eyed persons, patients living alone or unescorted, or those in whom medical problems arise during surgery).

Surgeons

Two ophthalmologists at all times   Residents and staff members

Surgical technique

100% intracapsular extraction   50% intra-capsular;
50% extra-capsular
selected in a randomized fashion with exceptions: high myopes, one-eyed patients, history of retinal detachment in either eye

Intra-capsular extraction

- Retrobulbar and akinesia (xylocaine 2%)
- Digital massage
- Limbal incision with Beaver blade
- Peripheral iridectomy
- Cryoextraction with a cryoextractor operated with freon gas
- A minimum of 10 8/0 Virgin Blue sutures
- Subconjunctival injection: gentamycin 20 mg and corticosteroid
  (Extra-capsular manual technique, without iridectomy)
- Metal eye shield

Follow-up (days)

- 1, 3, 7, and 21

Complications

- Minor complications (flattening of anterior chamber, pupillary block): ambulatory treatment (if possible)
- Major complications (wound dehiscence, iris prolapse, infection): hospitalize

Results: Day 21

- Anatomical success: yes or no
- Visual result: 20/40 or better
- (Spherical equivalent correction)—worse than 20/40

Surgical equipment and supplies

- Flash sterilizer
- 4 surgical instrument sets
- 1100 sutures
- Freon

– Surgical gowns, sheets, and gloves

Personnel

– 2 ophthalmologists
– 1 anesthesiologist
– 2 nurses
– 2 nurses' aids
– 2 stretcher bearers
– 1 cleaning aid

Travel (Chimbote only)

– 1 ophthalmologist, 1 nurse, 1 aid
– 25 round trips each
– 125 days per diem each

VIII. Management

The project will face a number of management problems. Not the least among these is securing government, community, and volunteer organization endorsement and contribution of project resources.

Another factor pivotal to each demonstration project is financial support. The proposed approach to demonstrating that a Cataract-Free Zone can be achieved introduces two unusual financial impacts: the cataract blind individual is not being asked to pay for medical services and, in attempting to clear the entire backlog of cataract blind cases, added costs are incurred beyond those associated with medical services. A funding agency must be sought if the projects are to be implemented as proposed.

The important next steps in the evolution of this proposal will be its review, with revision as appropriate, and validation by in-country personnel, that is, by individuals who will be involved in and affected by the project's implementation. Also, the detailed planning phases and development of the project's Manual of Operations will require a full time project co-ordinator, or operations manager. It is important that the recruitment of this individual be initiated soon. Funding for this individual and other planning-related costs must be obtained even before funding for project implementation is available. The co-ordinator's qualifications and duties are as follows:

A. *qualifications*

(1) Non-ophthalmologist.

(2) Regional/country person.

(3) On-site central location/office/vehicle.

(4) In-field survey experience.

(5) Operations management experience.

(6) 12-month commitment.

B. *Duties*

(1) Develop Manual of Operations.

(2) Documentation of communications.

(3) Overall co-ordination of project.

(4) Day-to-day monitoring.

The efficient day-to-day management of the project will be critical to its success, particularly since the implementation time frame is compact. Feedback and monitoring mechanisms must be developed to identify and rectify problems quickly before the integrity of the project is jeopardized. Project review meetings will need to be frequent and in-depth.

A planning timetable is shown. Using 15 April 1986 as a planning start date, it is estimated that the project will be ready for implementation after seven months of further planning and preparation (January 1987). The key pre-implementation activities are listed.

Planning timetable

	15 April 1986		Time in months		
	0	1.5	3	4.5	7
1. In country validation	|___|				
2. Obtain planning and pre-implementation support	|_____|				
3. Solicit community endorsement/involvement	|_____|			
4. Proposal finalization	|_____|				
5. Funding agency review		|_____|		
6. Project co-odinator recruitment	|_____|			
7. Prepare operations manual			|_____|	
8. Staff training				|_____|	

In similar fashion the proposed scheduling and duration of the components of implementation are diagrammed. Data analysis and project evaluation are shown as taking place over a three-month period, after all surgery and patient follow-up is completed

Implementation timetable

	January 1987 Start	2	Time in months 4	6	8	10	12
1. Mass Campaign	|_ _|__|						
2. Door-to-door survey	|_ _ _ _|_____|					
3. Eye examination	|_____|					
4. Surgery	|_____|					
5. Follow-up	|_____|					
6. Evaluation/data analysis					|_____|	

The proposed staffing of the project management team is as follows:

(a) Director (ophthalmologist): 20% for one year.
(b) Deputy Director (ophthalmologist): 20% for one year.
(c) Project Co-ordinator: 100% for one year.
(d) Secretary/administrative assistant: 100% for one year.

Organization chart

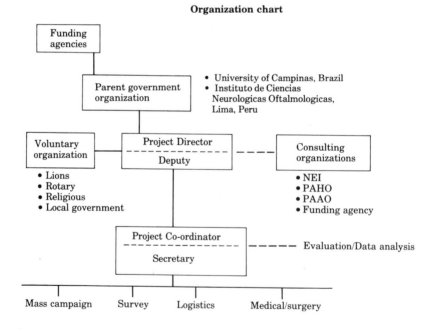

Attachment A: Participants in Planning Meeting

Pan-American Association of Ophthalmology, National Eye Institute, Fogarty International Centre, Meeting on Cataract-Free Zones, 1–4 April 1986, Stone House, National Institutes of Health, Bethesda, Maryland, USA

Joáo Fernando Berton, MD
Assistant Professor of
  Ophthalmology
University of Campinas
Rua Orlando Fagnani, Suite 157
13100 Nova Campinas
Campinas, São Paulo
Brazil

Vladimir Carazo, MD
Regional Advisor in Prevention of
  Blindness
Pan-American Health Organization
525 23rd Street, NW
Washington DC, 20037
USA

Francisco Contreras, MD
Hospital Santo Toribio de
  Mogrovejo
Laboratorio de Patologia Ocular
Ancash 1271
Lima
Peru

John Costello
Executive Director
Helen Keller International
22 West 17th Street
New York, NY 10011
USA

Leon Ellwein, Ph.D.
Associate Dean for Research and
  Development
University of Nebraska
College of Medicine
42nd and Dewey Avenue
Omaha
Nebraska 68105
USA

Edward A. Glaeser
Associate Executive Director
Helen Keller International
22 West 17th Street
New York, NY 10011
USA

Newton Kara-Jose, MD
Rua Prof. Artur Ramos, 183–8.°
  AND.
CEP 01454
São Paulo
Brazil

Jorge Litvak, MD
Chief, Division of Disease
  Prevention and Control
Pan-American Health Organization
525 23rd Street, NW
Washington DC, 20037
USA

Stephen J. Ryan, MD
Secretary-Treasurer/North of
  Panama
Pan-American Association of
  Ophthalmology and
Professor and Chairman
Department of Ophthalmology
University of Southern California
  School of Medicine
Doheny Eye Building
1355 San Pablo Street
Los Angeles
California 90033
USA

Michael Shwartz, Ph.D.
Associate Professor
Health Care Management Pro-
  gramme and

Operations Management
Department
School of Management
Boston University
621 Commonwealth Avenue
Boston
Massachusetts 02215
USA

Mr. Jack Swartwood
Helen Keller International
15 West 16th Street
New York, NY 10011
USA

Juan Verduguer, MD
Secretary-Treasurer/South of
   Panama
Pan-American Association of
   Ophthalmology
Luis Thayer Ojeda 0115
Oficina 305
Santiago
Chile

Craig K. Wallace, MD
Director
Fogarty International Centre
National Institutes of Health
Bldg. 38A, Rm. 605
9000 Rockville Pike
Bethesda
Maryland 20892
USA

Sir John and Lady Wilson
Impact
22 The Cliff
Roedean
Brighton
East Sussex
BN2 5RE
UK

NEI staff
Carl Kupfer, MD
Director
National Eye Institute
National Institutes of Health

Bldg. 31, Rm. 6A03
9000 Rockville Pike
Bethesda
Maryland 20892
USA

Edward H. McManus
Deputy Director
National Eye Institute
National Institutes of Health
Bldg. 31, Rm. 6A05
9000 Rockville Pike
Bethesda
Maryland 20892
USA

Roy C. Milton, Ph.D.
Head, Biometry Section
Biometry and Epidemiology
   Programme
National Eye Institute
National Institutes of Health
Bldg. 31, Rm. 6A16
9000 Rockville Pike
Bethesda
Maryland 20892
USA

Julian M. Morris
Associate Director for Programme
   Planning, Analysis, and
   Evaluation
National Eye Institute
National Institutes of Health
Bldg. 31, Rm. 6A27
9000 Rockville Pike
Bethesda
Maryland 20892
USA

Richard L. Mowery, Ph.D.
Health Scientist Administrator
Clinical Trials Branch
Biometry and Epidemiology
   Programme
National Eye Institute
National Institutes of Health
Bldg. 31, Rm. 6A24

9000 Rockville Pike
Bethesda
Maryland 20892
USA

Barbara A. Underwood, Ph.D.
Special Assistant to the Director
   for Nutrition Research and

International Programmes
National Eye Institute
National Institutes of Health
Bldg. 31, Rm. 6A08
9000 Rockville Pike
Bethesda,
Maryland 20892
USA

Attachment B: Decision diagram, from household search through 21-day follow-up

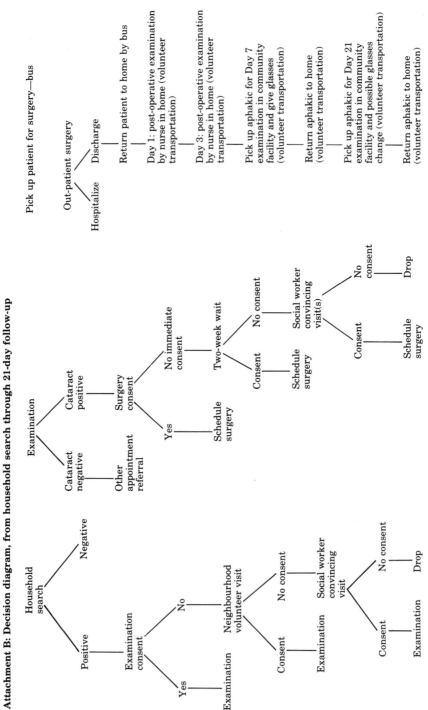

Appendix E

REPORT OF THE WHO INTERREGIONAL MEETING ON THE MANAGEMENT OF CATARACT WITHIN PRIMARY HEALTH CARE SYSTEMS *Denpasar, Indonesia, 15–19 December 1986*

CONTENTS

ιntroduction

An Interregional Meeting on the Management of Cataract within Primary Health Care Systems was convened in Denpasar, Indonesia, from 15 to 19 December 1986. The meeting was opened by H.E. the Governor of Bali, Professor I.B. Mantra, on behalf of the Government of Indonesia, and by Dr Suyono Yahya, Director-General of Community Health, on behalf of the Ministry of Health.

Professor Sugana Tjakrasudjatma was unanimously elected Chairman of the meeting, with Dr M.C. Chirambo as Vice-Chairman; Professor B.R. Jones was appointed rapporteur. The participants of this meeting included ophthalmological and public health experts from all WHO regions, together with a large number of representatives of international non-governmental organizations. The agenda, which was adopted without modification, is attached as Annex 1; the List of Participants will be found as Annex 2.

1. The magnitude of curable blindness due to cataract

1.1 General overview

Cataract was included as one of the main blinding disorders in the world in a resolution adopted by the World Health Assembly in 1975 (Resolution WHA28.54), but at that time no detailed information was available as to the magnitude of visual loss due to cataract. This condition is of particular importance, however, as it constitutes by far the most common cause of 'curable blindness', i.e. sight which can be restored by surgery.

When the WHO Programme for the Prevention of Blindness was established in 1978, increased attention was paid to cataract as a cause of loss of vision, together with the already well-known preventable causes, such as trachoma and xerophthalmia. Since 1980, a number of carefully conducted population-based surveys of blindness and its causes have invariably demonstrated that cataract is the leading cause of blindness. In virtually all recent epidemiological studies of blindness, cataract has been shown to be responsible for between a half and two-thirds of all blindness. If this proportion is applied to the estimated number of blind in the world (calculated to be 28 million in 1979), using the now internationally accepted definition of blindness as the inability to count fingers at a distance of 3 metres, it can be estimated that there are at present some 14 to 17 million blind due to cataract. A major proportion of these blind people could probably have their sight restored, were cataract surgery to be made available to all those in need of it.

Whilst developed countries have managed to control blindness due to cataract by providing adequate services for cataract surgery, the situation in most developing countries is different. The lack of facilities and scarcity of trained manpower have limited the provision of cataract surgery so that, in the majority of developing countries, there is an accumulating backlog of unoperated cases of blindness due to cataract. Furthermore, cataract surgery in these countries is usually confined to urban areas, thus leading to under-served rural areas, where the majority of the population is found. To this should be added the fact that cataract as a cause of visual loss is rapidly increasing in many developing countries, because of the growing proportion of the elderly in the population, cataract being closely related to age. There are also indications that blindness due to cataract may be more common and of earlier onset in some parts of the world, particularly in South-East Asia and possibly in Africa, which further adds to the problem of controlling blindness due to this disorder in many developing countries.

There is also an important time factor to be considered in making cataract surgery available to those needing it. Surgery must be provided within a few years of a cataract reaching maturity, in order to avoid complications, such as secondary glaucoma, which may lead to irreversible visual loss.

1.2 African region

There are no exact prevalence rates available for blindness and visual impairment in most African countries. However, based on results from some of the countries where population-based surveys have been conducted, the overall blindness rate for the Region is estimated to be 1 per cent to 1.5 per cent, thus giving a total of 6 million blind persons and about 24 million people with visual impairment.

Three million of these cases of blindness are due to cataract, which is curable were eye care facilities, trained personnel and financial resources to be made available. National committees for the prevention of blindness have been formed in almost all the countries of the Region. Not all the committees are active, but during the past decade some countries, in collaboration with the World Health Organization and non-governmental organizations, have developed and implemented national programmes for the prevention of blindness to address the major causes of blindness in general and cataract in particular.

In most countries, the cataract problem is being addressed within an incomplete framework of comprehensive eye care services. At the secondary and tertiary levels, ophthalmologists as well as non-ophthalmologists in certain countries provide cataract surgery. At the primary and community level, both mid-level health personnel and village health workers provide eye care services through primary health care systems.

The recent National Survey of Blindness and Blinding Disease in the Gambia demonstrated that in this West African country, with a population of approximately 800 000, there is a crude blindness rate of 0.7 per cent (age-adjusted rate of 1.7 per cent if compared to the United Kingdom). Untreated cataract accounts for 55 per cent of the blindness and comprises an estimated total of 5500 persons requiring cataract surgery. There is one ophthalmologist in government service.

1.3 Region of the Americas

The region is heterogenous: there are countries, such as Argentina, Chile, and Uruguay, that have a well-developed public health service that provides cataract surgery in such a way that no great cataract backlog exists, whereas in others, such as Brazil and Peru, a cataract backlog has accumulated. A survey in Bolivia of a representative village of 8000 inhabitants showed that the percentage of cataract blind was 0.6 per cent, representing the actual cataract backlog for that community.

In Brazil and Peru it is projected to create 'cataract-free zones' (Campinas and Chimbote respectively); these will involve a total population of over 100 000 being screened and operated as part of an operational research project in an effort to reduce the cataract backlog by 90 per cent. The success of this project will determine whether such a strategy can be replicated throughout the Region.

In North America, cataract surgery is a major activity of ophthalmologists. Because of the accessibility of these services there is little evidence for the existence of a cataract backlog of public health dimensions. From a cost perspective, however, cataract surgery represents a major expenditure of public health.

1.4 Eastern Mediterranean Region

Population-based data on cataract in the Eastern Mediterranean Region are only available from Saudi Arabia and Tunisia. A nation-wide stratified cluster random sample from the total population of Saudi Arabia, estimated to be around 9 million, was carried out in 1984. This showed cataract to be the leading cause of blindness (55 per cent of the total blindness), and the second leading cause of visual loss (35 per cent) after refractive errors.

In the age group 60 years and over, 64.5 per cent had significant cataract changes. In the age group 40 to 59 years, cataract was demonstrated in 24.5 per cent of cases, and in the age group 20 to 39 years, about 0.6 per cent were affected. There was no statistically significant difference in the prevalence of cataract among males and females. Cataract surgery had been carried out in 26.6 per cent of individuals with cataract, females having a lower rate of cataract surgery. Complications, unacceptable by modern standards, were demonstrated in 19 per cent of patients who underwent cataract surgery before 1984. Over 40 per cent of those operated still suffered visual loss owing to lack of proper spectacles. The rate of cataract surgery has improved dramatically during the last three years. It is estimated that 7000 operations are carried out annually in Saudi Arabia, over 4000 of which are performed at the King Khaled Eye Specialist Hospital. In a society that, on cultural grounds, shows a traditional aversion to using spectacles, the use of intraocular implants has enhanced the acceptability of cataract surgery.

A population-based survey was carried out in six central and southern gouvernorats of Tunisia in 1979 and 1980 to determine eye care needs. This survey was limited to the rural population, and included eye examinations of more than 8000 persons. The blindness rate was found to be 3.9 per cent and although trachoma was endemic in three of the six gouvernorats, cataract and its consequences contributed to visual loss in 60 per cent of cases.

In Jordan, cataract was found to be the leading cause of curable blindness in the West Bank and the Gaza Strip. Cataract has also been demonstrated to be the major cause of blindness in patients attending hospitals throughout the country.

1.5 *European Region*

Cataract surgery constitutes the main workload in ophthalmic units in Europe, and is provided through existing services. The actual dimension of unrecognized and unoperated cataract has not been determined.

1.6 *South-East Asia Region*

The South-East Asia Region, comprising 11 developing countries with a total population of over 1 billion, includes four countries in the least developed category with a joint population of nearly 120 million. Available epidemiological data show that the national prevalence rate of blindness ranges from a low of 0.2 per cent to nearly 2 per cent, with areas within some countries having blindness rates of up to 3 per cent. Population-based studies carried out in certain countries point to an average cataract prevalence accounting for over 50 per cent of all blindness. It is estimated that the backlog of cataract blindness in South-East Asia amounts to little under 8 million. The magnitude of the problem of blindness due to cataract and the urgent need for intensified action for sight-restoring intervention has to be viewed against the reported figure of 1.3 million cataract operations performed in 1985 in 9 of the 11 countries in the South-East Asia Region along with the anticipated absolute increase of the ageing population and age-related cataract in these countries over the next decade or so.

In India, according to a recent survey on the prevalence of cataract, it is estimated that there are 7.5 million eyes with mature and hypermature cataract and 2.4 million eyes with advanced immature cataract.

The clearance of the backlog of cataract is being effected on a priority basis by an active outreach 'eye camp' approach within primary health care services. All 'camps' are organized with the active participation of the community and in collaboration with voluntary organizations, ensuring equity of coverage. Trained ophthalmic assistants posted in Primary Health Centres assist in the investigation of cases of cataract, the maintenance of records and the organization of eye camps. The cost of surgery is being maintained at between US$10 and US$25, in addition to local input. Aphakic glasses costing from US$0.5 to US$1.0 are provided free of charge after surgery. Every effort is being made to ensure quality service, while the infrastructure is being strengthened to achieve a target of 2 million operations per year.

In Indonesia, epidemiological surveys have revealed that the prevalence rate of blindness is 1.2 per cent, of which 0.76 per cent of cases were of lenticular origin. This puts the number of persons blind from cataract-related causes at just under 1.5 million. The cataract backlog is estimated at over 1.25 million, all of whom are in need of surgery. The total number of aphakes in the whole country was estimated to be 142 000 in 1982. Since 1979, eye care and prevention of blindness programmes have been integrated into Primary Health Care systems. Since 1985 a pilot project on cataract relief services has been carried out in provinces of West Java, East Java, and Bali, to develop appropriate intervention methods, particularly in elaborating appropriate technology, and fostering community participation and intersectoral collaboration to eradicate the backlog of cataract.

The Nepal National Blindness Survey in 1980 and 1981 revealed that the second most prevalent condition next to trachoma was cataract. In total, an estimated 397 205 people (2.8 per cent of the population) were found with some degree of cataract. Of these, it was the primary disorder in an estimated 312 720 cases, and a secondary disorder in an additional 61 544 cases. Furthermore, there were 22 941 additional cases who suffered from cataract in which the lens had been surgically removed (aphakic), dislocated by couching or after cataract or other complications. Approximately 26 000 new cases of cataract blindness occur in Nepal each year.

In Sri Lanka, of the estimated 67 000 blind in both eyes, two-thirds, i.e. 46 000, are blind due to cataract. Out of this group of 46 000 people: 16 000 are between 60 and 70 years of age, and 9000 are over 70 years of age.

In Thailand, prevention of blindness based on a primary eye care approach was initiated in 1978. Activities are now being phased to integrate with Primary Health Care covering 30 provinces. A survey in 1983 disclosed an average blindness rate of 1.14 per cent, of which blinding cataract constituted 47.3 per cent, corresponding to 270 000 cases. The total number of cataract operations performed in 1985 is estimated at 20 000. A mass intervention scheme on a nation-wide scale has already been formulated based on the PHC approach. The field activities began in selected provinces in 1986, aiming at the creation of 'blinding cataract-free districts'. In addition to the service component, research activities are included in the operational plan at the provincial level.

1.7 Western Pacific Region

In an estimated total population of over 54 million in the Philippines, some limited surveys have suggested blindness rates of 2.6 per cent for the rural population, and 0.9 per cent for urban dwellers, with a national average of 2.13 per cent. Limited surveys in certain areas have suggested a national cataract prevalence of 1.1 per cent with rates of 4.35 per cent in a rural area and 0.59 per cent in urban Manila. The estimated backlog of cataract requiring operation is between 300 000 and 900 000 cases. The country has 195 ophthalmologists, of which 97 are based in Manila covering a population of 4.5 million. Most of the cataract in rural areas is being dealt with by ophthalmologists provided by non-governmental organizations.

No population-based data on blindness and/or cataract are available for the South-West Pacific. In Fiji, with a population of 700 000 scattered over 120 inhabited islands, some 600 cataract operations are performed per year. Control of the cataract backlog has been somewhat strengthened by the integration of primary eye care into the Fiji national primary health care programme. As the majority of qualified ophthalmologists are based in the urban areas, the rural population is under-served. The rural areas are mainly served by non-governmental organizations. In the other South-West Pacific nations, there are two ophthalmologists working in Western Samoa but no further information is available. The Solomon Islands, Tonga, Kiribati, Vanuatu, and Cook Islands have no local eye services other than the periodic clinics conducted by teams from Australia or New Zealand.

The major problems with eye care services in the South-West Pacific are:

(a) Relatively small national populations scattered over many islands.
(b) Low income and costly boat transportation making referral difficult.
(c) Understaffed medical systems depending on periodic eye clinics conducted by expatriates.

These nations need to be encouraged to be more self-sufficient in this respect.

In Vietnam, a long-standing trachoma control project has now been converted to include all categories of blindness control under a comprehensive national programme for the prevention of blindness. The primary health care approach is adopted as its key strategy. A recent survey disclosed that the blindness rate is 0.8 per cent of which 4.5 per cent are due to blinding cataract. A five-year programme recently formulated to identify five pilot areas (each of a population of 100 000), including the city of Ho Chi Minh, identified cataract for high priority action through the primary health care approach. The estimated cataract backlog is around 210 000 people. The annual cataract surgery output is about 5000 to 6000.

2. The public health problem of cataract blindness in developing countries

2.1 Introduction

The public health problem of cataract refers to ageing-related opacification of the crystalline lens of the eye, impairing vision to an extent that severely restricts occupational and/or other daily activities. This disorder, usually affecting both eyes, has a blinding propensity which, however, is amenable to surgical cure. The resulting blindness commonly constitutes a major public health problem in developing countries, where it needs to be tackled on a priority basis.

In addition to the usually bilaterally blinding cataract, some unilateral cases require early surgery to avert the threat of irreversible complications from hypermaturity of the cataract.

Bilateral congenital cataract is rare in comparison with age-related cataract, but does constitute an important component of blindness in childhood that needs early referral to secondary or tertiary eye care centres.

2.2 Epidemiology

By far the most common form of cataract relates to ageing. The vast majority of cataract blindness occurs beyond 50 years of age, but severe visual loss may occur between the ages of 40 and 50 years, or even earlier. In some countries it appears to be more common in females, but this may be a result of higher utilization of services for cataract surgery by males. It is important to include data on aphakia when reporting the prevalence of blindness from cataract.

The prevalence of cataract blindness accounts for half or more of the total blindness (in the absence of an additional burden of blindness from hyperendemic onchocerciasis or trachoma).

There is no proven means for preventing cataract blindness. Diabetes is undoubtedly a risk factor for cataract. Its increasing prevalence in certain parts of the world is a matter of concern, but diabetes cannot fully explain the public health problem of cataract blindness. A number of other possible risk factors have been advanced. The sunshine (or ultraviolet light exposure) theory of cataract formation is attractive but lacks definitive epidemiological support. Nutritional factors may be of relevance. Some studies have reported lower prevalence in communities living at high altitude than in lowland communities in the same countries, but other studies have showed the reverse. The relation between cataract and alcohol is also unclear. Episodes of severe dehydration from cholera-like diarrhoea, or heatstroke, may constitute an important risk factor for blinding cataract. These require further investigation in several geographical areas.

3. Strategies for action against cataract

In countries or regions where cataract blindness poses a problem of significant magnitude, intensified action needs to be taken to provide surgical cure and visual correction.

The strategies for such intervention might include:

- Assessment of the problem.
- Identification of cases.
- Creation of awareness in the population.
- Motivation of those blind to utilize services.
- Development of a referral system.
- Provision of cost effective surgical services to deal with large numbers.
- Provision of optical correction at an affordable cost.

The assessment of the problem is a necessary prerequisite not only for planning the setting up of services, but also for providing baseline data against which the impact of these services could be measured in subsequent evaluations. These assessments could be carried out by simple but epidemiologically sound data gathering. Involving the community in such assessments could also spur the community to take active part in the subsequent development of services. The identification of cases requiring referral for surgery must in the first instance rest with the community. This could be achieved through creating an awareness among the population of the condition and its potential for cure. Such identification, together with motivation of the affected person to utilize services, would help overcome some of the socio-cultural and behavioural constraints to acceptance of surgical treatment. The provision of adequate back-up services, particularly at the intermediate referral level and at outreach facilities, is a basic requirement to ensure credibility in community-based interventions. Such services should be developed and strengthened concurrently with the promotional activities at the community level.

In tackling the vast number of presently under-served persons blind from cataract the organization of cataract relief services on a large scale becomes of paramount importance. Because services may often need to be provided outside the precincts of the traditional eye care institutions, the organization of such services needs careful attention to detail, to ensure both safety and cost effectiveness.

The visual rehabilitation of the person after cataract surgery is perhaps as important as the surgery itself. The provision of aphakic spectacles at an affordable price or even free of charge should be ensured in the context of community-oriented services for cataract.

4. Application of cataract intervention schemes within primary health care

4.1 Case finding at community level

In many developing countries there is still a need to assess more accurately the magnitude of blindness due to cataract. Personnel at the primary health care level may assist in this endeavour, particularly community health workers, if properly trained. The health worker may carry out house-to-house visits in the search for blind people, and examine those found and establish a simple register, whilst arranging for their referral. The criteria for recognizing blindness presumably due to cataract must be quite simple at this level, the two most relevant criteria being:

- Visual loss (usually inability to count the fingers of a hand at a distance of 3 metres).
- White pupil.

Depending on the level of training of the health worker, it may also be possible to include the simple testing of pupillary reaction to light by means of a torch, and this should be carried out when feasible.

4.2 Referral

As a general referral instruction, in addition to visual loss and white pupil, the characteristics of a typical case of blindness due to cataract should be:

- Gradual loss of vision over several years without pain in an elderly patient.

In most situations, the health worker should be instructed to refer blind patients for further examination by more qualified personnel, to assess whether something may be done about the cause of blindness. This, however, presupposes adequate referral facilities; in any event, as a general rule for urgent referral within a primary eye care scheme, priority should be given to cases of sudden loss of vision and/or painful eyes.

One of the problems commonly encountered in the detection of individual cases of blindness due to cataract is the lack of awareness of the fact that cataract surgery may restore sight, and that this surgical procedure is safe and effective. Community health workers can, therefore, play a most important role in conveying this message to the local population, encouraging individuals with loss of vision to come forward for examination and possible referral for surgery. It is important that the health worker himself/herself has gained sufficient understanding about cataract as a cause of blindness, to ensure his/her co-operation and motivation to actively search for those cases, and to convince the community of the benefit in so doing. It should also be explained to the health worker that cataract is usually found in the elderly, and that the history of loss of vision is of importance.

In many countries, blind persons detected by the health worker will be referred to a health centre for further examination before being seen by a specialist for surgery. At the health centre level, more qualified personnel is normally available, such as nurses with some training in eye examinations, or in certain settings higher levels of staff including clinical officers and/or general physicians. At this level it is therefore usually possible to apply stricter diagnostic criteria for blindness due to cataract, to avoid the referral of too many cases of non-curable blindness due to other causes. The following may be tested at the health centre level in most settings:

- Visual acuity in each eye separately.
- Examination for projection of light.
- Absence or pronounced reduction of the red reflex, commonly together with a white pupil.
- Normal pupillary reaction to light stimulus.

In some cases, it may also be possible to measure intraocular pressure, provided a tonometer (normally Schiotz model) is available at the health centre, and that the personnel concerned has been sufficiently trained to obtain reliable readings. If these conditions apply, it is desirable to measure intraocular pressure in order to identify cases of obvious glaucoma with very high ocular tension before any surgery is considered.

4.3 Referral for surgery

The actual referral for surgery will depend not only on the patient's status, but also on access to the provision of cataract surgery. Here, it is of importance that overloading the referral system be avoided, that some kind of recording system be established for referral patients, and that there should be feedback from higher levels of eye care to the health workers at the community level.

As a normal procedure in most situations, there should be a written record, or special form provided for each referred case, giving the name, age, place of residence and date. It is also desirable that the reason for referral is given by the health worker, even if not necessarily as a clear-cut diagnosis, as this may also allow for an evaluation of his/her performance and possible need for further training. The feedback from the first referral, or higher, level should be arranged on a continuous basis, either by returning the referral forms with a brief description of action taken, or periodically in briefing sessions between the community health workers and the personnel at higher levels.

4.4 Factors to be considered for large-scale cataract surgery

To deal effectively with the public health problem of a massive backlog of cataract it is essential that safe and streamlined routines be established. These should include the continuing recruitment and training of staff to cover wastage. Other factors requiring consideration include the following:

Type of surgical procedure. There is general agreement that the safety, speed, and simplicity of the intra-capsular extraction under local anaesthesia makes it attractive and economic for the present purpose. Changing to the microsurgical technique of extra-capsular extraction would be dependent upon additional surgical skills and the availability of operating microscopes. Furthermore, it would incur a major decrease in surgical output and commonly requires a subsequent surgical procedure in the posterior lens capsule. The insertion of intraocular lenses would further complicate both the surgical procedure and the follow-up care. This would again reduce the number of cases operated upon and, in addition, increase the costs.

In any event, the wound should be closed with at least five fine sutures to reduce post-operative complications and allow for short hospitalization.

Allocation of adequate operating room space and time. In many situations the limit to surgical output is determined by insufficient availability of operating time and space. In others, the limiting factor is shortage of surgical instruments, drugs, and other materials. In these cases all means of overcoming the obstacle should be considered.

Team approach to the management of facilities and operating time. In most situations, the development of the team approach to the management of facilities and the flow lines in the surgical procedures will substantially increase the output that a given surgeon can maintain. The provision and training of adequate numbers of nursing and managerial staff in the team will free the surgeon from distracting tasks. Furthermore, it allows for the implementation of fail-safe surveillance routines to minimize the risk of breakdown of sterilization procedures and sterile techniques (see p. 168).

4.5 Follow-up procedures after cataract surgery

Cataract surgery may be carried out in a variety of local settings, such as regular eye departments, district hospitals, eye camps, or by the hospitalization of patients in temporary local wards set up for visiting mobile surgical teams. In all these various situations, the period of hospitalization and the arrangements for post-operative care of patients operated for cataract is of great importance. It appears that world-wide there is a general trend for shortened periods of hospitalization for cataract surgery, with an increasing amount of out-patient cataract surgery being performed in the most developed countries. In the setting of developing countries and rural populations there are, however, several factors to be taken into consideration:

- the surgical technique must provide a good wound closure to prevent complications in early mobilization of the patient;
- the patient must be able to comply with the post-operative treatment prescribed;
- the patient should normally be available for a daily post-operative assessment for a few days, with a subsequent final examination and provision of spectacles;
- the patient's social and economic status, together with transport problems, may necessitate a certain period of hospitalization.

It seems that, in many developing countries, a period of 5 to 7 days of hospitalization after cataract surgery is the present rule. There are, however, also examples of shorter periods (3 days) in some countries, but the possible risks of this shortened hospitalization have not yet been fully investigated, in terms of rate of complications or visual outcome. It is, nonetheless, of great importance that such studies be arranged, as a shortened period of hospitilization may allow a significant increase in the numbers of cases operated, provided there is capacity available for more cataract surgery in the locality concerned. This matter should, therefore, be considered a priority for operational research, to increase the output of cataract surgery within existing resources (see p. 167).

Post-operative treatment of cataract patients usually includes mydriatics, antibiotics, and often also topical corticosteroids. Personnel at the primary health care level may assist in the provision of such treatment, or the surveillance of patients under treatment.

4.6 Monitoring

In some situations it may be possible and useful to involve health workers or staff at health centres in the monitoring of possible post-operative complications, such as signs of infection or sudden visual loss. This may form part of a system for quality control of the services provided, i.e. an overall assessment of useful vision in operated patients, and its appreciation by the local community. It is of particular importance that every opportunity be taken to enable patients who are experiencing the benefits of cataract surgery to spread this information around in the local setting.

In all events, a system for the recording of complications during and immediately following cataract should form part of the system for provision of cataract surgery. This should preferably be done in a systematic and standardized manner, with regular analysis to permit identification of particular complications, and also to assess the performance of the responsible surgeon or surgical team in the local setting. It is of importance that quality control also be carried out on an independent basis, preferably by the appropriate professional organization.

4.7 *The provision of spectacles*

Following surgery for cataract, arrangements should be made for patients to obtain spectacles for optimal restoration of sight. This, unfortunately, poses a great problem in many developing countries, where spectacles are often hard to find and are excessively expensive. The following preliminary measures may be taken to remedy this situation:

(a) Cheap and effective technology is available for the local assembly of spectacles from imported, or locally accessible, lenses and frame components. This may be arranged by establishing local optical workshops, where a simple set of tools for the surfacing and cutting of lenses and for the fitting of lenses into frames can easily be arranged at low cost. Bulk import of standardized spectacle components may further reduce the cost. The workshop may employ two or three trained technicians, and may be set up as part of a hospital or eye department, or through local nongovernmental organizations. The training period for the technicians is usually around six to eight weeks.

The setting up of optical workshops, as described, has been successfully achieved in a number of countries, particularly in Africa. The initial investment required is approximately US$15 000 to US$20 000, including an initial stock of spectacle components. It has been demonstrated that spectacles may be produced in this way at a cost of US$3 to US$6, and a small profit may be included to make the system economically viable.

It has also been shown to be useful to involve the Ministry of Finance and/or the Ministry of Commerce in such a venture, as frequently the materials and equipment required can then be imported duty free.

(b) Spectacles may be bought at modest prices from some countries, e.g. India, and then imported into the country concerned. This system may pose problems with respect to the need for foreign currency, and the often high import duties on spectacles. Furthermore, this does not promote the future self-reliance of the importing country.

(c) In countries where there is an existing industry for the production of lenses and frames, it has sometimes been possible to reduce the cost by bulk purchase, and by requesting special prices on a welfare basis, to be used for local assembly of spectacles for operated cataract patients who could not normally afford to buy spectacles.

(d) It may be possible in certain countries to involve the optical industry and opticians in making available spectacles at reduced prices on a special prescription basis for poor patients. This would require consideration of the existing market, in order to ensure co-operation of all parties involved.

(e) Used spectacles or frames may be available as gifts from certain welfare organizations in developed countries. This, however, requires much work to measure all the lenses and classify them accordingly. There is also often the problem of unsuitable correction for astigmatism and anisometropia. Thus, even if the cost may be less for these spectacles, it should be seen as a temporary measure for small-scale projects.

Provision must also be made for the repair of broken spectacles, and to replace lost or scratched lenses. This is again usually most easily arranged in local optical workshops. Standardized frame models would facilitate the repair and replacement of spectacles, but attention must also be paid to the consumers' acceptance of spectacle models and shape of lenses.

5. Manpower resources and training of personnel

In most countries with an existing backlog of unoperated cases of cataract, there is a serious shortage of trained personnel to deal with the problem. This particularly refers to the availability of cataract surgeons, and this cadre of personnel must be dramatically and rapidly increased to permit the implementation of large-scale cataract intervention schemes in many countries.

There are, in general, four options for increasing the availability of cataract surgeons in a country:

(a) Increase the number of trained ophthalmologists who could assume responsibility for cataract surgery. This would require considerable investment in teaching facilities, and it would only have an impact several years later, in view of the long training period for the specialist level in most countries. Shorter periods of training, such as for a Diploma in Ophthalmology, would ensure the availability of suitably trained manpower to meet the immediate needs within a shorter time-frame. Such training courses, with emphasis on cataract surgery, need to be particularly encouraged and supported to increase the number of qualified ophthalmologists in a number of countries especially in Africa. Nevertheless, an increase in the number of qualified ophthalmologists is badly needed in a number of countries.

(b) Increase the number of cataract surgeons within the existing cadre of ophthalmologists in a country. Often only relatively few ophthalmologists are performing cataract operations in substantial numbers, while the majority perform very little or no surgery. It should be possible to involve more fully the national ophthalmological societies in cataract programmes, mobilizing their members to take a more active part in cataract surgery. This may be arranged on a periodic basis with voluntary work in rural areas, as part of a mobile team, or in fixed settings. Furthermore, more cataract surgery may be performed as part of the duties of junior ophthalmologists who may be posted in under-served areas for a given period.

(c) Increase the number of cataract operations by training new cadres of medical personnel to perform cataract surgery, such as general surgeons or medical officers. Training in cataract surgery may be arranged on an intense training programme basis for periods of 3 to 12 months, depending on previous surgical experience. This option allows a rapid increase in the number of cataract surgeons in a country, and may also facilitate the posting of such surgeons to rural areas.

(d) Training of paramedical personnel, such as ophthalmic assistants, to perform cataract surgery. This proposal is of interest to countries with an acute shortage of trained specialists, but with a rapidly growing backlog of cases of unoperated cataract, such as several countries in the African region.

It is clear that each country will decide on its own policy for prescribing qualifications for a cataract surgeon, but the use of general practitioners/surgeons or medical assistants for this purpose is already in place in some countries with positive results.

6. Community involvement and support

The need for community involvement and participation in eye health-related activities cannot be over-emphasized. Such participation should be actively promoted and fostered by providing information and education on the magnitude of the problem of blindness due to cataract in the community and on the curable nature of the condition. In this regard the perceptions of the community should be ascertained and taken into account when planning and implementing interventions.

In most developing countries, traditional medical practitioners are often not only respected members of the community but also serve as the front-line health providers for a large section of the community. Their active support and involvement could facilitate the delivery of cataract relief services. In mobilizing their support, it is necessary to impress upon them the disastrous effect of such procedures as couching for cataract. Provided with appropriate information and education on eye health, traditional medical practitioners could be a potent force in the motivation of the community and in fostering community acceptance of cataract relief services and greater compliance to treatment. As well as motivating the community to become involved, it would be necessary to identify resources from within the community itself, or from outside, to support the activities planned. Local organizations or philanthropic individuals can often be stimulated into providing support, and examples of such benefactors abound in some countries. Both the direct and indirect costs of surgery vary widely from country to country, and it is considered desirable to compute these costs at a country level using a standardized budgetary format (see Annex 3 p. 174).

Non-governmental organizations, both national and international, continue to provide technical and financial support to cataract relief services. In fact, the greater proportion of cataract operations in many developing countries is being carried out with varying support from non-governmental organizations which have indeed often pioneered action in this field, leading to subsequent governmental involvement and support. The basic strategy of non-governmental organization support should be to encourage the development of indigenous skills and self-reliance over an appropriate period of time. National resources should be gradually built up so as to sustain these activities even after international non-governmental organization support is withdrawn.

The WHO Programme for the Prevention of Blindness collaborates closely with several international non-governmental organizations active in providing cataract relief services in a number of developing countries. Further information on the work of these non-governmental organizations is available in the reports of the meetings of the WHO Programme Advisory Group on the Prevention of Blindness and the reports of the meetings of the Consultative Group of Non-governmental Organizations to the WHO Programme for the Prevention of Blindness. Copies of these reports are available on request from the PBL Office at WHO Headquarters, 1211 Geneva 27, Switzerland.

7. Co-ordination with other health programmes

Health care of the elderly and rehabilitation provide two examples of health programme areas which have a direct impact on blindness prevention programmes in general and cataract intervention in particular. Visual impairment has been identified as one of the more common health problems in the elderly. Besides impeding both domiciliary and self-care, visual disabilities impair the quality of life of this population group and detract from the independence, self-esteem, and the standing of the elderly in the community.

National blindness prevention programmes can establish mutually beneficial linkages with programmes for the health of the elderly in countries where these are active and this could also involve linking up with other non-governmental organizations.

The programme for rehabilitation of the disabled has increasingly reoriented towards both prevention of disability and community-based rehabilitation services for the disabled.

Such programmes are currently operational in several countries, often with non-governmental organization support, and include community-based screening for identifying disabled persons and their referral for treatment. Ophthalmological linkages with the rehabilitation programme at national levels should be encouraged.

8. Role of operations research in prevention of blindness activities

The term operations research has been used in a variety of ways with different meanings. Very simply defined, it is a methodology for problem definition, analysis and solution-seeking that considers all the relevant components and their interrelationships. The relevant components include environmental, economic, social, and behavioural factors. Operations research within the context of the community applies the scientific method to problem solving in the management and control of community systems using an interdisciplinary team approach in order to best serve the interests of the community as a whole. At the community level, this methodology should be carried out involving maximum community participation. Implicit in this definition is using the appropriate technology that will reach the largest number of individuals affected by the problem, considering how the chosen technology will have an impact on relieving of the problem in relation to available community resources. Further, the definition implies that the scientific method, i.e. definition of the problem, identification of causes and modelling of the potential solutions and evaluation of results, will be applied within the context of the communities' available resources or access to necessary resources at reasonable cost. Hence, operations research is very appropriate as a methodology within the concept of the primary health care system to address causes and solutions to public health problems. The backlog of curable age-related cataract blindness is, of course, one such public health problem.

The first task is to define the problem of blindness properly within the community setting its dimensions, consequences, causes, characteristics, social dimensions, and deterrents to solutions. This must be done at the local level since there is no universally applicable community programme for prevention of these blinding conditions that adequately considers, for example, cultural, social, and economic diversity.

Once the problem is defined, a careful analysis and modelling of cause and solution must follow. For the backlog of age-related cataract, only an increase in the number of operations will solve this component of the community blindness problem but there may be many different barriers to accomplishing this. These must be identified and the possible means of overcoming them considered.

Once a community analysis of the problem, its causes and potential solutions has occurred, the next step is to determine from the communities' perspective what the objectives of a specific programme to prevent blindness should be. If community leaders have been involved in the definition and analysis of the problem and its component parts, they will be better able to conceptualize how the problem fits into their total programme of community development and as a result set out precise, realistic goals or objectives for prevention of blindness activities. Based on these objectives, a careful analysis of available community resources must follow and be considered in balance with those available to meet overall community needs. Finally, the probable impact of the prevention of blindness programme decided upon relative to the needs of the community as a whole should be articulated as a basis for future evaluation.

In summary, operations research provides a strategy or methodology for planning, implementing, and evaluating prevention of blindness activities most of which can be carried out within communities with minimal external assistance. Importantly, those activities that do require external professional, logistical or economic aid can be clearly identified and justified.

In 1986, an international group of experts and representatives of nongovernmental organizations met to discuss issues surrounding the global conquest of cataract blindness (*To restore sight—the global conquest of cataract blindness.* Helen Keller International Inc., 15 West 16th Street, New York, NY 10011, USA). The group identified a series of project areas they felt deserved priority attention, among which were a series of operations research projects. These included research:

– to identify and motivate the cataract-blind to seek surgery;
– to improve access to cataract;
– to develop mimimum-level surgical facilities;
– to improve operating room efficiency;
– to reduce post-operative hospitalization; and
– to increase the number of ophthalmic personnel.

It is hoped that research projects in these areas within the context of the primary health care system will receive priority consideration.

9. Evaluation of cataract intervention schemes

Monitoring and evaluation of cataract intervention services should be an important in-built component of the planning for this activity. While monitoring would provide information on a day-to-day basis on the implementation of the scheme in relation to the planned time-frame, evaluation would indicate the achievement of the activity in relation to identified indicators and targets.

Monitoring should include an 'early warning system' to alert the team manager of any untoward complication that might point to a serious breakdown in the established delivery system or sterile surgical technique.

Evaluation should take stock not only of the quantity of services provided but also their quality and costs. Such analysis should be made available at short periodic intervals to the providers of services to enable them to improve their performance as well as to encourage them in their work.

Long-term evaluation may assess the unmet needs in the community in relation to cataract blindness, the impact of the intervention on the eye health status of the community and the well-being of the population. The evaluation should also include an assessment of coverage by the services, and of available resources including trained manpower and infrastructure.

Evaluation assumes particular importance in the context of non-governmental organization-supported activities both for the establishment of an acceptable accountability for resources provided and to facilitate their future fund-raising efforts.

Conclusions and recommendations

The participants of this Interregional meeting, having reviewed and discussed the following facts:

- that cataract is by far the most common cause of blindness in all countries, usually responsible for some 50 to 70 per cent of all blindness;
- that there are no proven preventive measures against the development of cataract;
- that loss of sight due to cataract can be successfully restored through surgery, and that such surgery is safe, effective and can be carried out at low cost; and
- that there is a growing backlog of unoperated cases of cataract reaching public health dimensions in many developing countries.

The participants wish to put forward the following conclusions and recommendations:

1. The magnitude and serious public health problem of blindness due to cataract has been demonstrated in a number of developing countries in recent years, including the existence of a backlog of unoperated cases. There is still, however, a need to assess this problem in other countries; it is, therefore, recommended that this be done as a matter of some urgency to allow for the planning and implementation of intensified action, within national programmes for blindness prevention, for large-scale provision of cataract surgery.

2. It is recommended that a primary health care approach be applied in countries to deal with cataract blindness, particularly for the early detection and referral of cases in need of surgery. These activities should be integrated into existing primary health care systems. In most of the countries concerned it will be necessary to allocate increased resources to overcome the problem of blindness due to cataract, which should form part of the development of general health services at the national level.

3. Whereas at the primary health care level measures to detect and refer cases of cataract in need of surgery can be introduced relatively easily, it will be necessary in many countries to strengthen the intermediate level of eye care, in order to perform a sufficient number of cataract operations. It is recommended that all possible means be sought to achieve this, making use of all applicable options to provide cataract surgery on a large scale, at

an accessible distance, and at low cost; options to be considered in this context may include mobile surgical teams, rural eye clinics, eye camps, and in certain areas fixed facilities for high-volume cataract surgery.

4. It is of great importance to promote awareness about cataract surgery and its benefits in afflicted communities, in order to encourage patients to come forward for operation. It is, therefore, recommended that measures be taken in the countries concerned, to spread information and education about cataract as a cause of curable blindness, and that communities are fully aware of and involved in local cataract intervention schemes. It is of particular importance that community health workers and personnel at the primary health care level are correctly informed and well motivated to participate in the promotion of cataract surgery.

5. It is strongly recommended that spectacles for aphakic correction be provided as part of the services for cataract surgery. This will allow optimal restoration of sight and at a modest cost if local schemes for the provision of spectacles at an affordable price are developed simultaneously. Governments should be encouraged to set up or facilitate the establishment of appropriate schemes to ensure that spectacles are made available at affordable cost to all patients operated for cataract.

6. One of the recognized constraints in many countries to gaining acceptance of cataract services has been the cost of surgery and corrective glasses. It is recommended that, while appropriate improvement in managerial and technological skills be adopted to reduce costs, resources be mobilized from the local community and national and international nongovernmental organizations to subsidize the cost of surgery and aphakic spectacles.

7. The professional ophthalmological organizations and academia should be oriented to the national priority for provision of adequate and appropriate surgical services for cataract. It is recommended that targets for t e number of cataract operations per annum should be set in countries with a substantial backlog in need for surgery.

8. There is a serious shortage of ophthalmologists in most developing countries. The length and cost of many existing training programmes are such that it is unlikely that these programmes can meet the needs of the countries concerned within the foreseeable future, given existing resource constraints. Additional shorter training schemes should be developed focusing on the needs of surgical services, while maintaining other educational schemes to meet the needs of academia. Governments should assume the responsibility for creating posts and career structures for the personnel thus trained.

9. In some countries, much of the general preventive and curative services are provided by personnel who are trained as clinical officers, through an extended apprenticeship. Certain of these are selected for training including cataract surgery. The quality of their cataract surgery has been

shown to be fully acceptable. It is recommended that this pattern be encouraged in countries where the need exists, and where national regulations so permit.

10. The training of personnel for the intermediate level of referral between the primary health workers and the secondary eye care level is recommended. Such personnel can play a vital role in training and supervising peripheral workers in eye health care and the recognition and referral of patients for cataract surgery.

11. Traditional healers play a very important role in providing information, or misinformation, about health, and in referral or non-referral of patients for scientific medical care. In many societies they act as front line health care providers. Their potential role in eye health education should be strengthened. They should be informed about the availability and effectiveness of cataract surgery and discouraged from harmful procedures, particularly couching.

12. There is a great need to use operational research as an effective tool to overcome obstacles to the provision of cataract surgery effectively, on a large scale, and at the lowest possible cost. It is recommended that studies in this respect be conducted in selected countries, including fields such as the consumers' and providers' behaviour in relation to utilization of health services, surgical techniques for optimal safety and cost, management of surgical wards and hospital facilities, and shortened hospitalization.

13. One important aspect of cataract surgery on a large scale is to ensure and maintain a system for quality control. It is recommended that this be included from the outset of national programmes addressing blindness due to cataract. Appropriate records of surgery provided, of complications, if any, and visual results, together with a simple but adequate follow-up reporting system should be developed to this end, involving health personnel at the primary health care level.

14. It is recommended that national programmes including cataract relief services be carefully monitored, and periodically evaluated against established targets. It is of particular importance that progress made be measured against the reduction of any existing backlog of unoperated cases.

15. As part of the search for preventive measures, it is recommended that further research on risk factors for cataract be conducted, with a view to identifying possible environmental or biological determinants, amenable to intervention.

16. It is recommended that every opportunity be taken to measure the impact on eye health, and in particular on cataract, that may result from the implementation of various components of primary health care.

Annex 1: Draft agenda

Opening of the Meeting
Election of Officers
Adoption of the Agenda

1. The magnitude of curable blindness (global and regional assessments)
2. Definition and epidemiology of blinding cataract.
3. Strategies for action against cataract
4. Application of cataract intervention schemes within primary health care:

    – case-finding,
    – assessment/referral,
    – referral for surgery,
    – follow-up procedures,
    – provision of spectacles,
    – quality control.

5. Training of personnel in relation to management of cataract
6. Community involvement and support
7. Co-ordination with other programme areas (care of the elderly)
8. Health systems research needs
9. Evaluation of cataract intervention schemes

Conclusions and recommendations
Closure of the Meeting

Annex 2: List of participants

Dr Marcelo Arze, Head, Teaching Department, Instituto Nacional de Oftalmología, Ministerio de Previsión Social y Salud Pública, Casilla No. 8011, La Paz, Bolivia.

Dr Ihsan Badr, Deputy Medical Director, King Khaled Eye Specialist Hospital, P. O. Box 7191, Riyadh 11462, Saudi Arabia.

Dr M. C. Chirambo, Principal Ophthalmologist, Ministry of Health, Kumuzu Central Hospital, P. O. Box 149, Lilongwe, Malawi.

Dr V. G. Hawley, Coordinator, Primary Eye Care Unit, Ministry of Health, Government Buildings, Suva, Fiji.

Dr Houang Thi Luy, Director, Dien Bien Phu Hospital, Ho Chi Minh City, Vietnam.

Professor Barrie R. Jones, former Director, International Centre for Eye Health, Department of Preventive Ophthalmology, Institute of Ophthalmology, 27/29 Cayton Street, London EC1V 9EJ, UK.

Professor Madan Mohan, Dr Rajendra Prasad Centre for Ophthalmic Sciences, All-India Institute of Medical Sciences, Ansari Nagar, New Delhi 110016, India.

Professor R. K. Radjamin Tamin, Head, Ophthalmological Department, Medical Faculty, Airlangga University, J1 Dharmahusada 8, Surabaya, Indonesia.

Professor Fuad Sayegh, Dean, Faculty of Medicine, University of Jordan, Amman, Jordan.

Dr Vicharn Srisupan, Eye Department, Buriram Hospital, Buriram, Thailand.

Professor Sugana Tjakrasudjatma, Director, Directorate of General and Teaching Hospitals, Ministry of Health, Jakarta, Indonesia.

REPRESENTATIVES OF NON-GOVERNMENTAL ORGANIZATIONS

Christoffel-Blindenmission (Headquarters: Nibelungenstrasse 124, D-6140 Bensheim 4, Federal Republic of Germany).

Dr Ronaldo A. Paraan, President, Project LUKE—Christian Healing Ministries, Inc., 505 National Life Insurance Co. Building, Session Road, Baguio City, Philippines 0201.

Helen Keller International Inc. (Headquarters: 15 West 16th Street, New York, NY 10011, USA)

Mr William Flumenbaum, Director, Nutritional Blindness Prevention and Control, Helen Keller International Inc., 15 West 16th Street, New York, NY 10011, USA.

Ms Donna Nagar, HKI Indonesian Programme Office, Jalan Jambu 40, Jakarta Pusat, Indonesia.

Dr Evangeline Olivar-Santos, Philippines Eye Research Institute, PGH Compound, Taft Avenue, Manila, Philippines.

International Agency for the Prevention of Blindness (Headquarters: National Eye Institute, National Institutes of Health, Building 31, Room 6A03, Bethesda, Maryland 20892, USA).

Dr Barbara Underwood, Special Assistant for Nutrition Research and International Programmes, National Eye Institute, National Institutes of Health, Building 31, Room 6A08, Bethesda, Maryland 20892, USA.

International Eye Foundation (Headquarters: 7801 Norfolk Avenue, Bethesda, Maryland 20814, USA).

Mr Jack Swartwood, Director, Programme Management, International Eye Foundation, 7801 Norfolk Avenue, Bethesda, Maryland 20814, USA.

Royal Commonwealth Society for the Blind (Headquarters: Commonwealth House, Haywards Heath, West Sussex, RH16 3AZ, UK).

Mr Alan Johns, Executive Director, Royal Commonwealth Society for the Blind, Commonwealth House, Haywards Heath, West Sussex, RH16 3AZ, UK.

174 *Appendix E*

SECRETARIAT

Dr G. Bambang Hamurwono, Chief, Sub-Directorate for the Prevention of
   Blindness, Directorate-General of Community Health, Ministry of
   Health, Jakarta, Indonesia.
Dr K. Konyama, Ophthalmologist, Programme for the Prevention of
   Blindness, World Health Organization, Avenue Appia, 1211 Geneva 27,
   Switzerland.
Mr H. L. Monga, Office of the WHO Representative, PO Box N 302, Jalan
   Thamrin, 14, Jakarta–46392, Indonesia.
Dr N. V. K. Nair, Regional Adviser for Nutrition, WHO Regional Office for
   the Western Pacific, PO Box 2932, Manila 2801, Philippines.
Professor A. Nakajima, Director, Department of Ophthalmology,
   Juntendo University School of Medicine, 3-1-3 Hongo Bunkyo-ku,
   Tokyo, Japan. (Temporary Adviser to the Secretariat).
Dr R. Pararajasegaram, Regional Adviser for the Prevention of Blindness,
   WHO Regional Office for South-East Asia, World Health House,
   Indraprastha Estate, Mahatma Gandhi Road, New Delhi 110002, India.
Dr M. Sathianathan, WHO Representative, PO Box N 302, Jalan
   Thamrin, 14, Jakarta 46392, Indonesia.
Dr B. Thylefors, Programme Manager, Programme for the Prevention of
   Blindness, World Health Organization, Avenue Appia, 1211 Geneva 27,
   Switzerland. (Secretary of the Meeting).

Annex 3: Management cost of cataract in India

Cost of maintenance of a blind person	US$ 0.50 per day
Costs due to loss of production	US$ 0.50 per day
Total loss per day	US$ 1.00
Total loss per year	US$365.00
Cost of restoration of sight to cataract blind	US$ 25.00

COST OF CATARACT SURGERY

	Paying ward patient	General ward patient
In tertiary care centres	US$150–US$200	US$40–US$50
In secondary care centres	US$40–US$50	US$20–US$25
In eye camps		US$22–US$28

(Inclusive of local inputs and cost of cataract glasses. Input made by local community in terms of volunteers and donations made in kind.)

Data provided by Professor Madan Mohan, Adviser in Ophthalmology,
Government of India

Index

175